SETON HALL UNIVERSITY

3 3073 00045644 0

D0559438

RESPONDING TO DISASTER

A GUIDE FOR
MENTAL HEALTH PROFESSIONALS

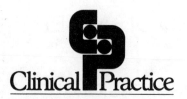

Clinical Practice

Number 24
Judith H. Gold, M.D., F.R.C.P.C.
Series Editor

RESPONDING TO DISASTER

A GUIDE FOR
MENTAL HEALTH PROFESSIONALS

Edited by

Linda S. Austin, M.D.

Associate Professor of Psychiatry
Director, Program for Public Education in Mental Health
Medical University of South Carolina
Charleston, South Carolina

SETON HALL UNIVERSITY
McLAUGHLIN LIBRARY
SO. ORANGE, N. J.

American Psychiatric Press, Inc.
Washington, DC
London, England

Note: The authors have worked to ensure that all information in this book concerning drug dosages, schedules, and routes of administration is accurate as of the time of publication and consistent with standards set by the U.S. Food and Drug Administration and the general medical community. As medical research and practice advance, however, therapeutic standards may change. For this reason and because human and mechanical errors sometimes occur, we recommend that readers follow the advice of a physician who is directly involved in their care or the care of a member of their family.

Books published by the American Psychiatric Press, Inc., represent the views and opinions of the individual authors and do not necessarily represent the policies and opinions of the Press or the American Psychiatric Association.

Copyright © 1992 American Psychiatric Press, Inc.
ALL RIGHTS RESERVED
Manufactured in the United States of America on acid-free paper
First Edition
95 94 93 92   4 3 2 1

American Psychiatric Press, Inc.
1400 K Street, N.W., Washington, DC   20005

RC
451.4
.D57
R47
1992

Library of Congress Cataloging-in-Publication Data
Responding to disaster: a guide for mental health professionals /
    edited by Linda S. Austin. — 1st ed.
        p.   cm. — (Clinical practice ; no. 24)
    Includes bibliographical references and index.
    ISBN 0-88048-464-0 (alk. paper)
    1. Disaster victims—Mental health services.   2. Disaster
victims—Mental health.   3. Crisis intervention (Psychiatry)—
Case studies.
    I. Austin, Linda S., 1951–   . II. Series.
    [DNLM: 1. Community Mental Health Services.   2. Crisis
Intervention.   3. Disaster Planning.   W1 CL767J no. 24 / WM 30
R4355]
    RC451.D57R47   1992
    362.2′04251—dc20
    DNLM/DLC   91-44366
    for Library of Congress   CIP

British Library Cataloguing in Publication Data
A CIP record is available from the British Library.

To Jerry, Stephanie, and Matt

Contents

Contributors

George W. Arana, M.D.
Professor of Psychiatry, Medical University of South Carolina, Charleston, South Carolina

Linda S. Austin, M.D.
Associate Professor of Psychiatry and Director, Program for Public Education in Mental Health, Medical University of South Carolina, Charleston, South Carolina

Andrew Baum, Ph.D.
Professor, Department of Medical Psychology and Department of Psychiatry, Uniformed Services University of the Health Sciences, Bethesda, Maryland

James Black, M.D.
Associate Clinical Professor of Psychiatry, Parkland Memorial Hospital, Dallas, Texas

Mel Blaustein, M.D.
Assistant Clinical Professor of Psychiatry, University of California, San Francisco, San Francisco, California

Etta C. Bryant, M.D.
Assistant Clinical Professor of Psychiatry, University of California, San Francisco, San Francisco, California

Raquel E. Cohen, M.D., M.P.H.
Professor, Department of Psychiatry, University of Miami Medical School, Miami, Florida

Alan R. Cole, M.D.
Psychiatrist in private practice, and Chair, Public Information Committee, Northern California Psychiatric Society, San Francisco, California

Hal Currey, B.S.
Administrator, Department of Psychiatry and the Behavioral Sciences,
Medical University of South Carolina, Charleston, South Carolina

Laura Davidson, Ph.D.
Research Assistant Professor, Department of Psychiatry, Uniformed
Services University of the Health Sciences, Bethesda, Maryland

Spencer Eth, M.D.
Assistant Professor of Psychiatry, University of California, Los
Angeles; and Clinical Associate Professor of Psychiatry, University of
Southern California, Los Angeles, California

Peter Forster, M.D.
Associate Clinical Professor of Psychiatry, University of California,
San Francisco, San Francisco, California

Lynda Frattaroli, M.S.W.
Associate Professor of Public Administration, College of Notre Dame,
Belmont, California

John R. Freedy, Ph.D.
Instructor of Psychiatry and the Behavioral Sciences, Medical
University of South Carolina, Charleston, South Carolina

John R. Gillette, M.D.
Associate Clinical Professor of Psychiatry, College of Osteopathic
Medicine of the Pacific, Pomona, California

Haikaz M. Grigorian, M.D., F.A.P.A.
Associate Professor of Clinical Psychiatry, University of Medicine and
Dentistry of New Jersey, Newark, New Jersey

Elizabeth Huggins, R.N., Ph.D.
Director of Nursing, Institute of Psychiatry, Medical University of
South Carolina, Charleston, South Carolina

Joyce C. Jarvis, M.P.A.
Executive Director, Northern California Psychiatric Society, San
Francisco, California

Dean G. Kilpatrick, Ph.D.
Professor of Psychiatry, Medical University of South Carolina,
Charleston, South Carolina

Susan Lynn McCammon, Ph.D.
Associate Professor of Psychology, East Carolina University,
Greenville, North Carolina

Lesly Tamarin Mega, M.D.
Professor of Psychiatry, East Carolina University, Greenville, North
Carolina

Lynn E. Ponton, M.D.
Associate Adjunct Professor of Child and Adolescent Psychiatry,
University of California, San Francisco, San Francisco, California

Jackie Puckett, A.C.S.W.
Project Administrator, Mobile Crisis Program, Medical University of
South Carolina, Charleston, South Carolina

Heidi S. Resnick, Ph.D.
Assistant Professor of Psychiatry and the Behavioral Sciences, Medical
University of South Carolina, Charleston, South Carolina

Harvey L. Ruben, M.D., M.P.H.
Associate Clinical Professor of Psychiatry, Yale University School of
Medicine, New Haven, Connecticut

Lenore C. Terr, M.D.
Clinical Professor of Psychiatry, University of California, San
Francisco, San Francisco, California

Joseph J. Zealberg, M.D.
Assistant Professor of Psychiatry and the Behavioral Sciences, Medical
University of South Carolina, Charleston, South Carolina

Introduction
to the Clinical Practice Series

O ver the years of its existence the series of monographs entitled *Clinical Insights* gradually became focused on providing current, factual, and theoretical material of interest to the clinician working outside of a hospital setting. To reflect this orientation, the name of the Series has been changed to *Clinical Practice*.

The Clinical Practice Series will provide books that give the mental health clinician a practical, clinical approach to a variety of psychiatric problems. These books will provide up-to-date literature reviews and emphasize the most recent treatment methods. Thus, the publications in the Series will interest clinicians working both in psychiatry and in the other mental health professions.

Each year a number of books will be published dealing with all aspects of clinical practice. In addition, from time to time when appropriate, the publications may be revised and updated. Thus, the Series will provide quick access to relevant and important areas of psychiatric practice. Some books in the Series will be authored by a person considered to be an expert in that particular area; others will be edited by such an expert, who will also draw together other knowledgeable authors to produce a comprehensive overview of that topic.

Some of the books in the Clinical Practice Series will have their foundation in presentations at an annual meeting of the American Psychiatric Association. All will contain the most recently available information on the subjects discussed. Theoretical and scientific data will be applied to clinical situations, and case illustrations will be utilized in order to make the material even more relevant for the practitioner. Thus, the Clinical Practice Series should provide educational reading in a compact format especially designed for the mental health clinician–psychiatrist.

Judith H. Gold, M.D., F.R.C.P.C.
Series Editor
Clinical Practice Series

Clinical Practice Series Titles

Treating Chronically Mentally Ill Women (#1)
Edited by Leona L. Bachrach, Ph.D., and Carol C. Nadelson, M.D.

Divorce as a Developmental Process (#2)
Edited by Judith H. Gold, M.D., F.R.C.P.C.

Family Violence: Emerging Issues of a National Crisis (#3)
Edited by Leah J. Dickstein, M.D., and Carol C. Nadelson, M.D.

Anxiety and Depressive Disorders in the Medical Patient (#4)
By Leonard R. Derogatis, Ph.D., and Thomas N. Wise, M.D.

Anxiety: New Findings for the Clinician (#5)
Edited by Peter Roy-Byrne, M.D.

The Neuroleptic Malignant Syndrome and Related Conditions (#6)
By Arthur Lazarus, M.D., Stephan C. Mann, M.D., and Stanley N. Caroff, M.D.

Juvenile Homicide (#7)
Edited by Elissa P. Benedek, M.D., and Dewey G. Cornell, Ph.D.

**Measuring Mental Illness: Psychometric Assessment
for Clinicians (#8)**
Edited by Scott Wetzler, Ph.D.

Family Involvement in Treatment of the Frail Elderly (#9)
Edited by Marion Zucker Goldstein, M.D.

Psychiatric Care of Migrants: A Clinical Guide (#10)
By Joseph Westermeyer, M.D., M.P.H., Ph.D.

Office Treatment of Schizophrenia (#11)
Edited by Mary V. Seeman, M.D., F.R.C.P.C., and
Stanley E. Greben, M.D., F.R.C.P.C.

The Psychosocial Impact of Job Loss (#12)
By Nick Kates, M.B.B.S., F.R.C.P.C., Barrie S. Greiff, M.D., and
Duane Q. Hagen, M.D.

New Perspectives on Narcissism (#13)
Edited by Eric M. Plakun, M.D.

**Clinical Management of Gender Identity Disorders in
Children and Adults (#14)**
Edited by Ray Blanchard, Ph.D., and Betty W. Steiner, M.B., F.R.C.P.C.

Family Approaches in Treatment of Eating Disorders (#15)
Edited by D. Blake Woodside, M.D., M.Sc., F.R.C.P.C., and
Lorie Shekter-Wolfson, M.S.W., C.S.W.

Adolescent Psychotherapy (#16)
Edited by Marcia Slomowitz, M.D.

Benzodiazepines in Clinical Practice: Risks and Benefits (#17)
Edited by Peter P. Roy-Byrne, M.D., and Deborah S. Cowley, M.D.

Current Treatments of Obsessive-Compulsive Disorder (#18)
Edited by Michele Tortora Pato, M.D., and Joseph Zohar, M.D.

Children and AIDS (#19)
Edited by Margaret L. Stuber, M.D.

Special Problems in Managing Eating Disorders (#20)
Edited by Joel Yager, M.D., Harry E. Gwirtsman, M.D., and
Carole K. Edelstein, M.D.

Suicide and Clinical Practice (#21)
Edited by Douglas Jacobs, M.D.

Anxiety Disorders in Children and Adolescents (#22)
By Syed Arshad Husain, M.D., F.R.C.P.C., F.R.C.Psych., and
Javad Kashani, M.D.

Psychopharmacological Treatment Complications in the Elderly (#23)
Edited by Charles A. Shamoian, M.D., Ph.D.

Responding to Disaster: A Guide for Mental Health Professionals (#24)
Edited by Linda S. Austin, M.D.

Psychiatric Aspects of Symptom Management in Cancer Patients (#25)
Edited by William Breitbart, M.D., and Jimmie C. Holland, M.D.

**Madness and Loss of Motherhood: Sexuality, Reproduction, and
Long-Term Mental Illness (#26)**
Edited by Roberta J. Apfel, M.D., M.P.H., and Maryellen H. Handel, Ph.D.

Treatment of Adult Survivors of Incest (#27)
Edited by Patricia L. Paddison, M.D.

**Rediscovering Childhood Trauma: Historical Casebook and Clinical
Applications (#28)**
Edited by Jean M. Goodwin, M.D., M.P.H.

Foreword

*T*his excellent and timely collection of clinical accounts and over-view of disaster intervention draws together the experience of a wide range of clinicians who have worked in many disaster settings. Such firsthand and practical descriptions will do much to provide a framework for those who are increasingly faced with the complex and stressful task of providing mental health care in response to such emergencies.

The last decade has seen the rapid development of a knowledge base about the mental health consequences of disaster and also of a wider experience of disaster intervention. Studies such as those of Shore et al. (1986) and McFarlane (1987, 1988) have highlighted the psychiatric consequences that may follow major disasters. Detailed studies such as those of the Scandinavian disaster research workers (Holen et al. 1983; Weisaeth 1983, 1989) have highlighted the traumatic impact of particular stressor components.

Models of mental health care intervention have been proposed for some time (Cohen and Ahern 1980; Raphael 1975, 1986; Wilson and Raphael, in press). As indicated in this volume, the initial scene of the disaster is one of great chaos, and the mental health professional may be called on to fulfill many supportive and practical roles while assessing and counseling individuals, families, and groups. The aims of intervention are first humanitarian and compassionate and then preventive, involving the provision of care and treatment where these are required. As indicated in the descriptions provided in this volume, shelters, school-rooms, hotels requisitioned for the purpose, and the bedside of the injured are among the many sites where such care may be provided.

The rationale behind emergency interventions depends on models such as those outlined in Chapter 1. Psychologically based treatments predominate, with the goal of mitigating the effects of the various traumas that individuals and groups have experienced during the disaster. Such traumas include the threat or perceived threat to one's own life or the lives of loved ones; encounters with the gruesome, mutilating, horrific, or massive deaths of others; loss of loved ones, property, or other resources; dislocation from home or community; personal injury or the

injury of loved ones; and responsibility trauma when an individual feels
that he or she contributed to or somehow did not prevent someone else's
injury or death. Other aspects are also at times traumatic, or perceived so,
and this individual perception needs to be understood and worked with
by the clinician. Reactions during the emergency period may also be
important, including dissociation, failure to act in ways that the individual felt he or she should act, and cognitive distortions of time or perceptions occurring as a result of the trauma. Some individuals who are
precipitated into the "disaster syndrome" may need protection until their
stunned and apathetic state lessens and they can reorient to reality. The
importance of supporting and reuniting family members and of ensuring
adequate information sources so that victims may find or be found by
other loved ones is also very relevant.

The individual or team providing mental health care needs to be able
to assess those contacted in early intervention and outreach programs, to
document relevant issues and care, to identify those at risk, and to ensure
ongoing service provision for those whose difficulties may require more
intensive or prolonged treatment.

As Cohen and Ahern (1980) so clearly identified, mental health
professionals must also link carefully with the mental health care systems
of the community affected by the disaster. This can involve forming a
consortium with them or providing consultative services, ensuring adequate resources, and directing the victims to providers of traditional
services, when appropriate.

It is a sad commentary that after almost two decades of intervention
in disaster and widespread recognition of the importance of this intervention, the effectiveness of such intervention has rarely been evaluated.
Singh and Raphael (1981) showed some positive effects of a bereave-
ment-based intervention program after a rail disaster, but systematic and
comparative models of research-based assessment and intervention have
not yet been uniformly applied. It is important that sensitive and systematic care provision such as that described in this volume includes assessment of the effects of such actions on outcome—how these actions are
perceived by those who experience them and their impact on the prevention of posttrauma morbidity. Clearly, controlled trials are not possible in
such circumstances, but dose-response effects of both trauma and intervention can contribute to the knowledge of vulnerability and its modification and may be helpful in providing a basis for intervention in future
catastrophes.

A number of authors of chapters in this volume have commented on the stresses experienced by those providing such emergency care. This warrants special attention. One should develop the capacity to recognize and deal with one's own reaction to death, destruction, and loss; the reawakening of one's own earlier traumatic experiences; one's fears; and the deeper and chaotic aspects of one's own mind. As is highlighted here, countertransference issues may be very powerful. These may range from the "counterdisaster syndrome" of compulsive overinvolvement to the distancing of detachment and avoidance. It is important for disaster workers in the field to maintain the capacity for compassionate warmth and human involvement, yet at the same time not become overinvolved.

The rationale for emergency intervention rests on models such as those of military psychiatry (Solomon and Benbenishly 1986)—in which proximity, immediacy, and expectancy are the principal parameters—and of crisis intervention (Caplan 1964). Similar principles also underlie the processes of debriefing, in which opportunities are provided for emergency workers and others exposed to extreme stress to work through the traumatically stressful aspects of their work. Here, too, there is a need for evaluation.

This volume is invaluable in its descriptions of real-life, hands-on experience and the ways in which clinicians have adapted their knowledge and skills to provide for those affected by disasters. Described are innovative approaches ranging from the use of a "libidinal cocoon" to classroom consultation. All are likely to be helpful and are geared to an increasing understanding of responses to trauma in both children and adults. The disasters described are both "natural" (e.g., Hurricane Hugo) and "human-made" (e.g., Dallas airplane crash), and the clinical interventions are adapted to both. The disasters discussed are both small scale (e.g., Guadalupe River drowning) and large scale (e.g., Armenian earthquake), yet many common principles apply. The inescapable horror, the threat to life and loved ones, and the loss of home and community are all facts of disaster with which one must deal. This volume will be invaluable to all mental health professionals who are concerned with what to do when disaster strikes.

Beverley Raphael, M.D., F.R.A.N.Z.C.P., M.B.B.S., F.R.C.Psych.
Fellow, Australian Academy of Social Science
Corresponding Fellow, American Psychiatric Association
Professor and Chairperson, Department of Psychiatry,
University of Queensland, Queensland, Australia

References

Caplan G: Principles of Preventive Psychiatry. New York, Basic Books, 1964

Cohen RE, Ahern FL: Handbook for Mental Health Care of Disaster Victims. Baltimore, MD, Johns Hopkins University Press, 1980

Holen A, Sund A, Weisaeth L: Survivors of the North Sea oil rig disaster. Paper presented at the Symposium on Disaster Psychiatry, Stavanger, Norway, 1983

McFarlane AC: Post-traumatic phenomena in a longitudinal study of children following a natural disaster. J Am Acad Child Adolesc Psychiatry 26:746–769, 1987

McFarlane AC: The longitudinal course of post-traumatic morbidity: the range of outcomes and their predictors. J Nerv Ment Dis 176:30–39, 1988

Raphael B: Crisis and loss counselling following a disaster. Mental Health of Australia 14:118–122, 1975

Raphael B: When Disaster Strikes. New York, Basic Books, 1986

Shore J, Tatum E, Vollmer WM: Psychiatric reactions to a disaster: the Mt. St. Helens experience. Am J Psychiatry 143:590–595, 1986

Singh B, Raphael B: Post-disaster morbidity of the bereaved: a possible role for preventive psychiatry. J Nerv Ment Dis 169:203–212, 1981

Solomon Z, Benbenishly R: The role of proximity, immediacy, and expectancy in frontline treatment of central stress reaction among Israelis in the Lebanon War. Am J Psychiatry 143:613–617, 1986

Weisaeth L: The study of a factory fire. Unpublished doctoral dissertation, University of Oslo, Oslo, Norway, 1983

Weisaeth L: A study of the stressors and the post-traumatic stress syndrome after an industrial disaster. Acta Psychiatr Scand Suppl 355:25–37, 1989

Wilson J, Raphael B: The International Handbook of Traumatic Stress Studies. New York, Plenum (in press)

Preface

*T*he primary goal of this book is to provide a guide to organizing mental health services for a community traumatized by disaster. The first section covers general issues that should be considered after any disaster, including evaluation of the impact of the disaster on the community, prediction of the psychological sequelae of the disaster, and assessment of the cultural context of the disaster. In other chapters in this section, authors discuss general organizational issues of disaster response and the use of large-group interventions and media activities that are required to reach the stricken population.

The goal of the second section is to illustrate these issues and techniques with case reports of interventions and observations at particular disaster sites. The chapters illustrate that disaster responses must be individually planned according to the nature and intensity of the catastrophe and the characteristics of the population affected. The chapters in the second section reflect how the authors' responses were also shaped by their personalities and motivations. These motivations were quite diverse, reflecting spiritual, political, academic, and organizational concerns and affiliations. The concerns shaped the observers' perceptions of the disaster and became organizing influences as they established their priorities for organizing clinical services. It is my hope that the readers of this book will gain increased knowledge about mental health aspects of disasters and an appreciation of the significant emotional impact of serving a traumatized community.

Linda S. Austin, M.D.

Section I

Evaluating and Planning
a Clinical Response
to a Community Disaster

Chapter 1

Conceptual Framework for Evaluating Disaster Impact: Implications for Clinical Intervention

John R. Freedy, Ph.D.
Heidi S. Resnick, Ph.D.
Dean G. Kilpatrick, Ph.D.

*D*isasters are extremely complex events. Contemporary research and clinical workers categorize disasters as high-magnitude stressful life events (Baum 1987). This approach to disasters intuitively makes sense because it allows application of previous empirical work concerning stress, coping processes, and treatment approaches to important concerns regarding disasters. The viewpoint presented in this chapter is that empirical and clinical knowledge concerning the impact of disasters on individuals, groups, and communities has advanced to a stage that calls for the development of more sophisticated ways of thinking about disasters and their mental health impact.

Although disasters are stressful events, it is an oversimplification to view disasters as unitary events that affect all victims equally. In reality, disasters have more of an impact on some victims than on others. Furthermore, individuals differ in their capacity to adjust to the demands created by a disaster. In this chapter, we present a comprehensive framework for understanding the impact of various types of disasters. The major emphasis is on providing information relevant to

Preparation of this chapter was supported in part by National Institute of Mental Health Grant 1 T32 MH18869, Child and Adult Sexual Abuse: A Training Grant, and National Institute of Mental Health Grant 1RO1 MH47508-01A1, Disasters' Impact Upon Adults and Adolescents.

the planning of clinical assessment and treatment.

An initial requirement for any area of study is to define the nature of the phenomenon under consideration. Most broadly, disasters can be classified as either natural or technological (Baum 1987). Natural disasters considered in this volume include earthquakes, hurricanes, floods, tornadoes, and volcanic eruptions. Technological disasters considered in this volume include plane crashes, nuclear accidents, dam breaks, and toxic chemical spills. It can be stated, however, that any disaster characterized by the following elements is likely to disrupt individual and social functioning: powerful impact, low predictability, low controllability, threat, terror, and horror (Baum 1987; Gibbs 1989).

An additional requirement for any area of study involves establishing the substantial importance of the topic. This task is not difficult when considering disasters. First, disasters are common events. One illustration of the continual threat from disasters is the fact that, on average, 2.8 hurricanes impact the coastline of the United States each year (B. Case of the National Hurricane Center, personal communication, January 1990). Second, disasters affect large numbers of people. One estimate suggests that in each year from 1970 to 1980 approximately 2 million residents of the United States suffered injuries or property damage due to disasters (Solomon 1989). Third, no data suggest that disasters will occur less frequently or affect fewer individuals in the future. Experts have argued that factors such as increased population in coastal areas (vulnerable to hurricanes and flooding) and increasing technological complexity heighten the future risk of natural and technological disasters adversely affecting individuals (Baum 1987; B. Case, personal communication, January 1990). Fourth, disasters have been described as producing a range of notable psychological and physical dysfunction. The following reactions, ranging from mild to severe, have been associated with exposure to various disasters: posttraumatic stress disorder (PTSD), anxiety disorders, depression, psychosomatic complaints, substance abuse, brief reactive psychoses, and a range of aggressive behavior, such as domestic violence and arrests for intoxication (Gibbs 1989). Fifth, the dysfunctional reactions associated with disaster experiences can be persistent. Although emotional distress may dissipate in the weeks and months after a disaster (Cook and Bickman 1990), more persistent emotional reactions have been documented up to 5 years after a nuclear accident (Baum 1987; Baum et al. 1983) and 14 years after a dam collapse (Green et al. 1990).

Developing a Risk Factor Model

An optimal model for understanding disaster impact should specify the critical elements that determine who will adjust well and who will adjust poorly. The DSM-III-R (American Psychiatric Association 1987) diagnostic category of PTSD provides a meaningful starting point. This diagnostic category specifies a characteristic stress adjustment process by linking stressors "outside the range of usual human experience" (p. 250) to a pattern of reaction characterized by reexperiencing (e.g., nightmares), avoidance (e.g., mental or behavioral avoidance), and heightened arousal (e.g., hypervigilance). Although PTSD is not the only or even the most likely outcome from disaster exposure, the PTSD framework may be used as a heuristic device for identifying factors associated with different levels of postdisaster adjustment. Broadly speaking, this diagnostic category presents two principles that are critical in adjusting to any traumatic event. First, the importance of a time frame is implied. Factors existing before the stressor event (e.g., age, life experiences, previous emotional disorder), at the time of the stressor event (e.g., whether the event was caused naturally or by humans), and after the stressor event (e.g., environments resembling the original trauma) are recognized as potentially having an impact on the level of adjustment. Second, the importance of interactive mechanisms are implied. Characteristics of the individual (e.g., perceptions of threat) may interact with characteristics of the environment (objective nature of the stressor) across time in determining the level of adjustment (American Psychiatric Association 1987).

Consensus has emerged across combat, sexual assault, and disaster literatures concerning the types of factors important in determining mental health outcome after such events (Baum 1987; Foy et al. 1987; Green 1990). It appears that exposure to traumatic events can be associated with both acute and prolonged mental health difficulties (Green et al. 1990; Madakasira and O'Brien 1987). In addition, both objective (e.g., physical injury) and subjective (e.g., perception of life threat) facets of traumatic event exposure contribute to emotional distress (Kilpatrick et al. 1989). Most importantly, it is clear that not all individuals respond to traumatic events with the same pattern of adjustment. This latter fact suggests that individual differences with regard to mediating variables (e.g., social support, mental health history) may be very important in determining the course of individual adjustment after exposure to any traumatic event (Keane 1985).

In the remainder of this chapter, we devote attention to reviewing the current state of knowledge regarding the importance of exposure and mediating factors in determining adjustment after natural and technological disasters. Particular attention is given to providing this information in a manner that will help mental health professionals plan clinical interventions.

A Risk Factor Model of Disaster Adjustment

Consistent with earlier comments, we propose a model that recognizes the necessity of both a time frame and the interaction of a range of individual and environmental factors in predicting adjustment to disasters. Our proposed risk factor model is presented in Table 1–1. In the interest of clarity, the model will be discussed according to the chronology of the factors we propose as critical in determining disaster adjustment. In general, we propose that factors before a disaster, at the time of a disaster, and after a disaster interact to determine the emotional outcome experienced by any disaster victim. As shown in Table 1–1, we consider the following predisaster characteristics to be germane in influencing mental health outcome: demographic characteristics, high-magnitude life events, low-magnitude life events, history of mental

Table 1–1.   Risk factor model of disaster adjustment

• **Predisaster factors**	• **Postdisaster factors**
Demographic characteristics	Initial distress level
High-magnitude life events	Stressful life events
Low-magnitude life events	Resource loss
Mental health history	Coping behavior
Coping behavior	Social support
Social support	

• **Within-disaster factors**
　　Disaster exposure
　　Cognitive appraisal of
　　　disaster exposure
　　　　- Low control
　　　　- Low predictability
　　　　- High life threat

health problems, coping behavior, and social support. We propose that the following factors from the time of the disaster are important in determining postdisaster adjustment: disaster exposure and cognitive appraisal of exposure experiences (e.g., low control, low predictability, high life threat). We suggest that the following factors during the postdisaster period are important in determining emotional outcome: initial level of distress, stressful life events in the recovery period, social and personal resource loss related to stressful life events in the recovery period, coping behavior, and social support. The proposed model is a parsimonious representation of existing empirical data and theory concerning natural and technological disasters. We begin by reviewing information concerning factors present before disaster.

Predisaster Factors

Demographic characteristics. Gibbs (1989) reviewed empirical literature concerning the impact of demographic characteristics on postdisaster adjustment. Children are particularly vulnerable to experiencing emotional distress; findings concerning adults are mixed. It is not clear whether younger or older adults are most vulnerable to adjustment difficulties. Men and women appear equally affected by disaster when a broad range of psychopathology is considered. Women tend to express more emotional complaints (e.g., depression, anxiety), whereas men tend to display more substance abuse and other forms of problem-producing behavior. The findings are mixed with regard to social class. It seems plausible to suggest that individuals from less-advantaged socioeconomic groups are more vulnerable to psychological distress owing to difficulties in overcoming economic and physical hardships engendered by disasters.

Experiential factors. Several predisaster experiential variables may be important in determining postdisaster adjustment. The nature of life events experienced may have an impact on psychological and physical functioning. High-magnitude stress events of the type defined in criterion A of the DSM-III-R PTSD diagnosis (e.g., witnessing a violent death) may be associated with subsequent psychological and physical dysfunction. For example, research has documented that the victims of violent crime are prone to experience an alarming increase in rates of major mental health difficulties (Kilpatrick et al. 1985b,

1987a, 1987b). It is also likely that less intense life events (e.g., marital conflicts, financial difficulties) can be positively associated with psychological and physical distress (Lazarus and Folkman 1984). It may be that individuals faced with a high number of negative life events in the year prior to experiencing a large-scale disaster are vulnerable to subsequent adjustment difficulties.

Coping and social support. Research focused on the effect of predisaster coping behavior and social support on postdisaster adjustment is sparse. Accordingly, our comments are primarily derived from the general coping and social support literatures. Individual coping refers to a range of cognitive and behavioral efforts to solve problems, manage emotions, or disengage from difficult problems or painful emotions (Carver et al. 1989; Lazarus and Folkman 1984). A central task in coping is to differentiate threatening situations from benign circumstances, arranging one's responses accordingly. No single coping response is optimal in all situations. Rather, coping most likely produces optimal psychological and physical states when characterized by diversity and flexibility (Lazarus and Folkman 1984). It follows from this analysis that prior success experiences in coping with a range of life circumstances (e.g., employment, marriage, parenthood) should result in more confident attitudes regarding one's coping skills. However, this is disputed by Gibbs (1989), who reported that empirical findings do not support the belief that predisaster psychopathology predicts postdisaster adjustment.

Relationships are also central in maintaining psychological and physical adjustment (Hobfoll et al. 1990). Social support refers to both the perception of being socially connected and the functional exchanges (e.g., information, assistance on a task, emotional support) that occur between individuals (Hobfoll 1988). Similar to individual coping responses, there are instances when social support fails to enhance individual well-being (Hobfoll and Freedy 1990). For example, if relationships are dysfunctional (e.g., dependent relationships), the likely result is the perpetuation of negative psychological states (e.g., lowered self-esteem, frustration, resentment). Review of the complexities determining when social support is beneficial is beyond the scope of this chapter (see Hobfoll and Freedy 1990; Hobfoll et al. 1990). However, it is probably accurate to propose that individuals who were engaged in predisaster relationships that promoted personal control and competence possess an adaptive advantage over those not so richly endowed.

Within-Disaster Factors

Disaster exposure. Experiences occurring at the time of a disaster may be particularly relevant in determining the course of postdisaster adjustment. Green (1990) reviewed research concerning exposure to combat, disaster, and criminal assault. It was suggested that exposure to the following types of experiences was particularly salient in determining mental health outcome: threat to life or physical integrity, physical injury, receipt of intentional harm, exposure to grotesque sights, violent or sudden death of a loved one (witnessed or not), and information regarding exposure to a noxious agent. A sampling of disaster literature confirms that exposure factors appear causally related to subsequent psychological distress. For example, Green et al. (1990), reporting on the Buffalo Creek Dam flood in Buffalo Creek Valley, West Virginia, in February 1972, found that the following types of exposure factors were related to a range of PTSD symptoms up to 14 years after the flood: degree of exposure to the elements, loss of a household member, being blocked from escape, and being injured. One year after the May 1980 Mount Saint Helens volcanic eruption in southwest Washington State, individuals who had experienced high exposure (property loss or death of a close family member) were 11–12 times more likely to experience major depression, generalized anxiety disorder, or PTSD than individuals spared such experiences (Shore et al. 1986). Two to 4 months after the July 1985 Los Angeles, California, Baldwin Hills fire, residents at the scene of the fire experienced heightened PTSD symptoms, and those who lost their homes displayed significantly more depressive symptoms than residents who did not lose their homes (Maida et al. 1989). Exposure to the Three Mile Island nuclear accident 10 miles south of Harrisburg, Pennsylvania, in March 1979, particularly proximity to the reactor, has been associated with heightened symptoms of depression and anxiety at 17 months and up to 5 years (Baum 1987; Baum et al. 1983).

Cognitive appraisal or attributions. Perceptions of exposure experiences form an additional set of variables influencing disaster adjustment. Lazarus and Folkman (1984) are primary proponents of the position that perceptions of events are responsible for determining emotional and physical responses. Kilpatrick and Resnick (in press) reported that for crime victims in two community samples, the subjective perceptions of serious life threat and threat to physical integrity were positively associated with symptoms of PTSD. The relationship of these perceptual factors to emotional outcome was as strong as the relationship between objective physical injury and emotional outcome. Foa et al. (1989) reviewed cognitive variables related to PTSD. They suggested that to the extent an event was uncontrollable, unpredictable, or personally threatening, a poorer emotional outcome would result. Jones and Barlow (1990) also reported that perceptions of control, predictability, and threat were of particular importance in the development and maintenance of PTSD. They suggested that the tendency to maintain perceptions germane to a traumatic event beyond the time frame of the traumatic event (e.g., low control, low predictability, high threat) would heighten long-term emotional distress.

Postdisaster Factors

Acute experiences. Events occurring in the weeks and months after a disaster may also influence the level of adjustment. Here it may be helpful to distinguish between acute experiences and ongoing demands. Regarding acute emotional reactions, it is possible that intensity of initial emotional reactions predicts subsequent psychological distress. Kilpatrick et al. (1985a) reported that initial distress level was the best predictor from a set of variables in determining level of distress 3 months after a rape.

Ongoing experiences. Disasters often set into motion a series of ongoing stressful life events (e.g., job loss, residential displacement, separation from loved ones). Solomon and Canino (1990) examined the importance of disaster exposure and disaster-related life events in predicting symptoms of PTSD among victims of two disasters. The first sample of victims experienced flood and dioxin exposure in St. Louis, Missouri, in winter 1982. It was determined that exposure to the flood predicted the presence of a host of stressful life events. Furthermore, life events were of primary importance in predicting psychological distress 1 year after the flood. The second sample of victims, from Puerto Rico, experienced mud slides in October 1985. Exposure to mud slides and subsequent stressful events were both related to PTSD symptoms after 2 years, with three stressful events more strongly related to PTSD than exposure factors. Again, ongoing life events related to the disaster were more important in understanding psychological distress than the acute factor of disaster exposure.

Bereavement is a tragic life event that may accompany a disaster. The Armenian earthquake of December 1988 provides an extreme example, with more than 25,000 deaths. Most disasters are associated with less bereavement, although it remains an important concern. Wortman and Silver (1987) reviewed research concerning bereavement. It was concluded that the sudden, dramatic loss of a loved one (e.g., spouse, parent, child) is often associated with prolonged psychological distress. In fact, the emotional distress of bereaved individuals may remain significantly elevated compared with that of nonbereaved individuals up to 7 years after bereavement experiences. Typical reactions include depression, anxiety, somatic concerns, and impaired social functioning. Further, intense feelings concerning the loss can reemerge throughout the lifetime, particularly when cued by anniversaries and other reminders. In the case of disasters, bereavement is likely to be sudden and dramatic. Consistent with the proposed risk factor model, the inability to predict or control disaster-related bereavement should exacerbate psychological distress.

A contemporary stress theory, the Conservation of Resources (COR) model, can be applied to suggest why disaster-related life events produce psychological distress (Hobfoll 1989). The COR model focuses on the extent to which people maintain social (e.g., family roles, work roles) and personal (e.g., possessions, self-esteem, financial resources) characteristics that can be used to offset environmental demands. The model labels critical social and personal characteristics as resources. Resources, then, are tools that are useful in the process of successfully meeting a variety of environmental demands. The COR model proposes that negative psychological experiences result when environmental demands overwhelm available social and personal resources. The negative emotional experience resulting from unsuccessful resource investment is proposed to occur whether the resource loss is actual or perceived (Hobfoll 1988, 1989).

The breadth of the COR model makes it particularly applicable to understanding adjustment to life events in the postdisaster environment. The COR model specifies four broad resource categories: objects, conditions, personal characteristics, and energies. *Objects* are resources that are always external and possess both instrumental and appraised value. Examples of objects include home, car, and other possessions. *Condition* resources are external social ties and roles that provide both benefits and liabilities for the individual. Examples of conditions include marriage, parenthood, and employment. *Personal characteristics* are internal resources, based on the socially learned process of developing skills and attitudes regarding personal attributes. Examples of personal characteristics include self-esteem, self-efficacy, and sense of meaning or purpose. *Energies* are resources that are either internal or external and are valued as a commodity to be invested to accrue other resources. Examples of energy resources include money, time, and knowledge or skills (Hobfoll 1988).

The utility of the COR model in understanding adjustment to life events in the postdisaster environment is illustrated by applying the model to a hypothetical individual attempting to adjust after Hurricane Hugo devastated the Charleston, South Carolina, area in September 1989. (The authors of this chapter were direct victims of Hurricane Hugo.) Our disaster victim might experience a negative impact on the following resources after the storm: loss of shelter, loss of home contents, disruption in employment (with related financial and self-esteem difficulties), loss or disruption in social ties (permanent or temporary), threat to sense of control, loss of time, and loss of money. The COR model suggests that the attenuation of available resources will make it difficult for our disaster victim to meet the diverse and complex demands of life events following the hurricane. Faced with the threat of being unable to meet even basic needs due to insufficient social and personal resources (a basic human motive of self and social protection being compromised), the predictable result is acute psychological distress (Hobfoll 1988, 1989). Prolonged emotional distress will result if our victim cannot compensate for losses through individual, social, and community-wide efforts.

Several studies have begun to apply the COR model in an attempt to understand the adjustment of university personnel approximately 3 months after Hurricane Hugo. Individuals reporting more extensive aggregate resource loss (objects, conditions, personal characteristics, and energies) were significantly more likely to experience clinically elevated levels of psychological distress (Freedy et al., in press; Shaw et al. 1990). Further, aggregate resource loss was the strongest predictor of psychological distress (34.1% of distress variance), followed by demographic variables (9.5% of distress variance), and coping behaviors (7.9% of distress variance) (Freedy et al., in press). The primary importance of resource loss in predicting psychological distress after a hurricane highlights the importance of resource loss in predicting psychological adjustment during the postdisaster period. Additional evidence supporting the disruptive influence of resource loss following Hurricane Hugo includes the fact that extensive aggregate resource loss was associated with significant elevations in use of alcohol and prescription medicines (Jarrell et al. 1990) and significant disruptions in health maintenance behaviors, including diet, exercise, and weight changes (Bene et al. 1990).

Coping and social support. Consensus exists concerning the importance of coping efforts and social support in determining personal adjustment following disaster (Cook and Bickman 1990; Gibbs 1989). Gibbs reviewed the importance of coping behavior in mediating disaster impact and noted that existing studies do not allow definitive statements concerning the complex role of coping behavior. However, it was suggested that coping efforts resulting in a sense of control, sense of meaning, or emotional respite following disaster were beneficial. Cook and Bickman examined the role of social support in determining psychological adjustment following a flood and found that social support was not related to symptomatology immediately or at 5 months. However, social support and psychological symptoms were significantly related during the intermediate time period (1 week to 5 months), with those individuals low in social support experiencing significantly higher levels of psychological distress.

Comments concerning cultural influences on the efficacy of coping efforts and social support are speculative since disaster research seldom addresses cultural factors. Many cultural groups maintain strong kinship ties. Under routine circumstances, individual needs for coping assistance and social support are met within rather than outside of kinship networks (Stack 1974). The demands created during a disaster can be so massive that kinship networks are unable to meet all individual needs. At such times, reaching beyond community and kinship ties can be a source of distrust, embarrassment, or frustration (Lindy and Grace 1986). This may be especially true when reliance on an "outsider" is either profound or prolonged. It is likely that psychological distress after a disaster is reduced when disaster victims are able to rely on themselves with supplemental assistance from close kinship and community contacts. People from all cultures desire to support their own kin and to cope in such a way as to experience a sense of control, meaning, and emotional respite.

Assessment and Treatment of Disaster Victims

The information summarized in the proposed risk factor model suggests that the development of effective mental health assessment and treatment is important. As mentioned, disasters are common events that affect large numbers of people. Most notably, the range of psychological and physical dysfunction experienced by disaster victims can persist for months or even years after a disaster. At present, which disaster victims will adjust well and which will adjust poorly are not precisely understood. The risk factor model presented in this chapter represents a framework for more precisely predicting individual adjustment after a disaster. It is implicit in the risk factor model that adjustment to a disaster is a complex process unfolding over time, hence the emphasis on assessing characteristics of both disaster victims and their environment before, during, and after disaster impact. It is also implicit in the risk factor model that characteristics of the disaster victim (e.g., available social support) will interact with characteristics of the environment (e.g., postdisaster stressful life events) in determining level of postdisaster adjustment.

In the remainder of this chapter, we present assessment and treatment principles that are consistent with the proposed risk factor model.

Needs Assessment

An initial step in disaster preparedness involves prior planning. All communities are not equally vulnerable to all disasters. Therefore, it is critical that mental health service providers conduct thorough needs assessments regarding community vulnerability to various disasters. First, this involves making a list of natural disasters (e.g., earthquakes, hurricanes, tornadoes, flooding) and technological disasters (e.g., chemical spills, plane crashes, nuclear accidents) that may threaten a particular community. Second, it is important to consult reliable resources to determine the physical and psychological needs likely to be created by the disaster(s) in question. Examples of reliable information sources include this chapter and the other chapters of this volume, journal articles, and direct consultation with professionals from a community previously affected by the disaster under consideration. Third, plans must be made to meet the various physical and psychological needs likely to follow the disaster in question. This step may involve consultation with a range of professional groups, both mental health professionals and other groups (e.g., police, fire and rescue, churches), to ensure that adequate preparations are made to meet the diverse physical and psychological needs likely to arise after any disaster.

Our personal experience has been as both victims and service providers after Hurricane Hugo. Based on our experiences with Hugo, we offer two additional comments relevant to needs assessment and subsequent service delivery. First, catastrophic disasters require broadly based interventions. After Hurricane Hugo, there were important roles played by many service providers, including mental health professionals, police, fire and rescue workers, the Red Cross and other service organizations, government agencies, churches, media, and neighbors helping neighbors. No one individual or group can meet the diverse needs within a community of disaster victims. Second, intervention efforts should be targeted at multiple levels of needs, including individual, group, and community needs. Examples of individual-level interventions included crisis counseling at emergency shelters and neighbors helping neighbors to remove debris from homes. Examples of targeting group-level needs included providing stress management sessions to groups such as employees or church congregations and churches providing day care services to assist families struggling to recover. Examples of community interventions included media efforts to provide information and advice to the community and government-sponsored community-wide debris pickup services.

Role Boundaries

Prior to any disaster, most mental health professionals develop a workable balance between professional role demands (e.g., clinical service delivery) and personal role demands (e.g., being a spouse, parenthood). Catastrophic disasters absolutely disrupt existing professional and personal roles. For example, two of the three authors of this chapter were displaced from their homes for many months after Hurricane Hugo.

Under such circumstances, the primary task of the victimized mental health professional becomes meeting personal and family needs (e.g., shelter, food, clothing). The meeting of professional responsibilities often must be deferred to colleagues, temporarily, while personal needs are addressed. Alternatively, it is critical for mental health professionals engaged in service delivery to disaster victims to appreciate the intensity of their task. Most clinical workers have experience in addressing the needs of an individual trauma victim (e.g., a single rape victim, a bereaved father). After a disaster, clinical workers are faced with addressing the needs of hundreds or even thousands of trauma victims, including colleagues and family members. Therefore, it is advisable that clinical work be limited in time and that the professional engage in regular consultation with colleagues for support. Above all, it is important for the professional to set careful limits in balancing professional and personal responsibilities to promote both personal welfare and the quality of services provided.

Acute Interventions

Examination of the proposed risk factor model suggests the characteristics of individuals at high risk for adjustment difficulties in the days and weeks after a disaster. In particular, disaster victims who report high disaster exposure (e.g., threat to life, physical injury, exposure to grotesque sights), a certain pattern of cognitive appraisals (low control, low predictability, high threat), and intense initial emotional reactions may be at risk for intense and perhaps prolonged emotional turmoil. We recommend that clinical workers assess the presence or absence of each of these factors with a brief clinical interview. In addition, initial intensity of emotional reactions can be measured with one of several brief, statistically sound self-report measures. Examples of relevant instruments include the Symptom Checklist 90—R (Derogatis 1983), the Beck Depression Inventory (Beck and Steer 1984; Beck et al. 1961), the State-Trait Anxiety Inventory (Spielberger 1983), and the Impact of Events Scale (Horowitz 1986; Horowitz et al. 1979). The selection of an appropriate measure of psychological distress should be based on targeting the types of symptoms (e.g., depressed affect, anxious affect, somatic complaints) anticipated from the affected population.
    The model of stress debriefing provides a viable treatment modality immediately after catastrophic events (Mitchell and Bray 1990).

Adapted to the postdisaster environment, debriefings are structured meetings offered by mental health professionals for the benefit of potentially vulnerable individuals. These meetings can last 60–90 minutes and can be offered in settings where individuals typically gather (e.g., work sites, churches, community centers). It is important to bear in mind that many individuals are uncomfortable in seeking formal mental health services; therefore, it may be helpful to promote debriefings as stress-management sessions and not a formal psychotherapy group. For further discussion of debriefing techniques, see Forster (Chapter 2, this volume) and Cohen (Chapter 4, this volume).

Ongoing Interventions

It was suggested while describing the postdisaster phase of the risk factor model that disasters often set into motion a series of life events. In particular, it was suggested that the loss of a wide range of personal (e.g., home, self-esteem, money) and social (e.g., employment, social contacts) resources during the postdisaster period was largely responsible for subsequent adjustment difficulties (Freedy et al., in press). Recognition of the fact that ongoing life events and related resource loss constitute primary risk factors for later adjustment difficulties requires a conceptual shift in the focus of intervention efforts. Namely, it may be helpful for mental health professionals to conceptualize the postdisaster needs of victims in terms of a hierarchy of needs (Maslow 1968). First, efforts should be made to assist the victim in meeting basic physical and safety needs (e.g., shelter, food, water, clothing). Second, social needs might be addressed by making sure that the victim becomes reintegrated with previous social contacts (e.g., family, work, church). Third, needs related to self-evaluation (e.g., sense of control, self- esteem) could be addressed, but only after more basic physical and safety needs and social needs have been satisfied.

Our clinical approach following Hurricane Hugo involved a brief clinical interview to assess the presence or absence of various types of resource loss. To guide our questions, we used the 52-item Resources Questionnaire[1] modified from the Conservation of Resources inven-

---

[1]Available from the Crime Victims Research and Treatment Center, Department of Psychiatry and Behavioral Sciences, Medical University of South Carolina, 171 Ashley Avenue, Charleston, SC 29425-0742.

tory, developed by Hobfoll and colleagues (1991). We conceptualized the report of loss in terms of the previously mentioned hierarchy of needs. Some hurricane victims tragically lost their homes and most of their possessions. Assisting these victims in finding shelter and the like was not only functional, but provided these individuals with a sense of support and hope, thus reducing subsequent psychological distress. Some hurricane victims were more fortunate in that their homes and possessions were not destroyed. These individuals often expressed a compelling need to assist their neighbors and work colleagues to provide for basic needs. Interestingly, helping others appears to reduce the emotional distress of the helper. In terms of the hierarchy of needs, we suggest that by helping others, these victims were meeting their own needs for social connection and meaningful self-evaluation (e.g., control, purpose, self-esteem). It is our recommendation that mental health professionals provide an invaluable service by activating existing support systems. Whether through debriefing sessions, media-based education efforts, or other means, it is important that individuals and organizations within the postdisaster community be encouraged to assist all victims in meeting existing physical, social, and psychological needs.

The possibility exists that the intervention efforts described to this point might be insufficient to prevent the development of chronic psychological distress. Consider, for example, that the psychological distress persisting 3 months after a rape appears to remain stable 3 years after the rape (Kilpatrick 1985). A similar prognosis may apply to the pattern of psychological distress after other traumatic events, including disasters. We recommend, therefore, that more comprehensive treatment be considered for individuals who suffer from psychological distress that interferes with functioning at a point 3 months postdisaster. Stress inoculation training is an example of a comprehensive skills training approach that addresses cognitive, affective, and behavioral dimensions involved in persistently stressful circumstances (Meichenbaum 1985). Clinical and research data support the efficacy of this approach with rape victims (Foa et al. 1991; Kilpatrick and Amick 1985; Veronen and Kilpatrick 1983). Exposure-based techniques (e.g., flooding, systematic desensitization) with the goal of extinction of maladaptive affective, cognitive, and behavioral responses provide a second treatment alternative. Empirical data support the efficacy of exposure-based techniques (Fairbank and Brown 1987). Finally, treatment based primarily on cognitive restructuring might be offered to trauma victims (Foy et al. 1990). Although empirical evaluation of cognitive approaches are pending, conceptually this approach proposes to examine and change dysfunctional attitudes that may have developed in the wake of trauma (e.g., self-blame, low sense of control) (Janoff-Bulman 1985). For further discussion of intervention techniques for acute stress, the reader is referred to Terr (Chapter 5, this volume).

Mediating Factors

In closing our discussion of intervention principles, we return to the complex issue of predicting postdisaster adjustment. The predisaster and postdisaster sections of the risk factor model identify variables that are important in predicting postdisaster adjustment. We recommend that a brief clinical interview be used to assess predisaster and postdisaster factors within a developmental framework. With regard to predisaster variables, the following variables provide a basis for speculating about the course of postdisaster adjustment: high-magnitude life events, low-magnitude life events, and mental health history. To the extent that an individual has been successful in managing a range of life vicissitudes before a disaster, it is reasonable to expect that this individual possesses the social support, coping responses, and other resources necessary to adjust well following disaster. Conversely, individuals who have been unsuccessful in managing a range of life experiences before a disaster would be expected to be at risk for poorer postdisaster adjustment. Limitations on available social support, coping options, and other resources could further hamper efforts to adjust. A sensitive interview can inform the clinical worker concerning the diversity of each victim's capacity to meet disaster-related demands. Some victims will require little more than reassurance and encouragement to adjust well. Other victims will require extensive multidisciplinary efforts to meet their physical, social, and self-evaluation needs.

A developmental perspective can also be applied to postdisaster variables in predicting disaster adjustment. Here, it is important to question disaster victims regarding the life events and related social and personal resource loss they have experienced. Inventories such as the aforementioned Resources Questionnaire (Freedy et al., in press) or the Social Readjustment Rating Scale (Holmes and Rahe 1967) are useful guides in defining relevant life events and resource loss areas to assess.

It is important to assess jointly the available social support (e.g., family, friends, work colleagues) and the capacity to engage in required coping responses (e.g., financial losses uninsured). It would be predicted that disaster victims with both limited postdisaster life events and related resource loss coupled with available social support and coping options would adjust well following disaster. Conversely, disaster victims affected by serious postdisaster life events and related resource loss (e.g., loss of home, loss of job, bereavement) coupled with unavailable social support and limited coping options would experience adjustment difficulties.

The complexity of events determining adjustment during the postdisaster period highlight, once again, the individual nature of disaster impact and recovery. It is wise for the mental health professional to understand that by meeting the needs of disaster victims individually, the chances of optimal adjustment are maximized. This often requires efforts by both mental health professionals and other agencies and individuals to meet the diverse needs of individual disaster victims.

References

American Psychiatric Association: Diagnostic and Statistical Manual of Mental Disorders, 3rd Edition, Revised. Washington, DC, American Psychiatric Association, 1987

Baum A: Toxins, technology, and natural disasters, in Cataclysms, Crises, and Catastrophes: Psychology in Action. Edited by VandenBos GR, Bryant BK. Washington, DC, American Psychological Association, 1987, pp 9–53

Baum A, Gatchel RJ, Schaeffer MA: Emotional, behavioral, and physiological effects of chronic stress at Three Mile Island. J Consult Clin Psychol 51:565–572, 1983

Beck AT, Steer RA: Internal consistencies of the original and revised Beck Depression Inventory. J Clin Psychol 40:1365–1367, 1984

Beck AT, Ward CH, Mendelson M, et al: An inventory for measuring depression. Arch Gen Psychiatry 4:561–571, 1961

Bene CR, Jarrell PM, Shaw DL, et al: The disruption of health maintenance behaviors following traumatic stress: implications for clinical intervention. Poster presented at the 24th annual meeting of the Association for the Advancement of Behavior Therapy, San Francisco, CA, November 1990

Carver CS, Scheier MF, Weintraub JK: Assessing coping strategies: a theoretically based approach. J Pers Soc Psychol 56:267–283, 1989

Cook JD, Bickman L: Social support and psychological symptomatology following natural disaster. Journal of Traumatic Stress 3:541–556, 1990

Derogatis LR: SCL-90-R: Administration, Scoring and Procedures Manual—II, 2nd Edition. Baltimore, MD, Clinical Psychometric Research, 1983

Fairbank JA, Brown TA: Current behavioral approaches to the treatment of posttraumatic stress disorder. Behavior Therapist 3:57–64, 1987

Foa EB, Steketee G, Olasov-Rothbaum B: Behavioral/cognitive conceptualizations of post-traumatic stress disorder. Behavior Therapy 20:155–176, 1989

Foa EB, Olasov-Rothbaum B, Riggs DS, et al: Treatment of posttraumatic stress disorder in rape victims: a comparison between cognitive-behavioral procedures and counseling. J Consult Clin Psychol 59:715–723, 1991

Foy DW, Carroll EM, Donahoe CP: Etiological factors in the development of PTSD in clinical samples of Vietnam combat veterans. J Clin Psychol 43:17–27, 1987

Foy DW, Resnick HS, Carroll EM, et al: Behavior therapy with PTSD, in Handbook of Comparative Treatments. Edited by Bellack AS, Hersen M. New York, Wiley, 1990, pp 302–315

Freedy JR, Shaw DL, Jarrell MP, et al: Towards an understanding of the psychological impact of natural disasters: an application of the Conservation of Resources stress model. Journal of Traumatic Stress (in press)

Gibbs MS: Factors in the victim that mediate between disaster and psychopathology: a review. Journal of Traumatic Stress 2:489–514, 1989

Green BL: Defining trauma: terminology and generic stressor dimensions. Journal of Applied Social Psychology 20:1632–1642, 1990

Green BL, Lindy JD, Grace MC, et al: Buffalo Creek survivors in the second decade: stability of stress symptoms. Am J Orthopsychiatry 60:43–54, 1990

Hobfoll SE: The Ecology of Stress. New York, Hemisphere Publishing, 1988

Hobfoll SE: Conservation of resources: a new attempt at conceptualizing stress. Am Psychol 44:513–524, 1989

Hobfoll SE, Freedy JR: The availability and effective use of social support. Journal of Social and Clinical Psychology 9:91–103, 1990

Hobfoll SE, Freedy J, Lane C, et al: Conservation of social resources: social support resource theory. Journal of Social and Personal Relationships 7:465–478, 1990

Hobfoll SE, Lilly RS, Jackson AP: Conservation of social resources and the self, in The Meaning and Measurement of Social Support: Taking Stock of 20 Years of Research. Washington, DC, Hemisphere Publishing, 1991

Holmes TH, Rahe RH: The social readjustment rating scale. J Psychosom Res 11:213–218, 1967

Horowitz MJ: Stress Response Syndromes, 2nd Edition. Northvale, NJ, Jason Aronson, 1986

Horowitz M, Wilner N, Alvarez W: Impact of Events Scale: a measure of subjective distress. Psychosom Med 41:209–218, 1979

Janoff-Bulman R: The aftermath of victimization: rebuilding shattered assumptions, in Trauma and Its Wake. Edited by Figley CR. New York, Brunner/Mazel, 1985, pp 15–35

Jarrell MP, Bene CR, Freedy JR, et al: Normative alcohol and medication use patterns following a natural disaster. Poster presented at the 24th annual meeting of the Association for the Advancement of Behavior Therapy, San Francisco, CA, November 1990

Jones JC, Barlow DH: The etiology of posttraumatic stress disorder. Clinical Psychology Review 10:299–328, 1990

Keane TM: Defining traumatic stress: some comments on the current terminological confusion (letter). Behavior Therapy 16:419–423, 1985

Kilpatrick DG: The sexual assault research project: assessing the aftermath of rape. Response to the Victimization of Women and Children, Journal of the Center for Women Policy Studies 8(4):20–24, 1985

Kilpatrick DG, Amick AE: Rape trauma, in Behavior Therapy Casebook. Edited by Hersen M, Last CG. New York, Springer, 1985, pp 86–103

Kilpatrick DG, Resnick HS: PTSD associated with exposure to criminal victimization in clinical and community populations, in Posttraumatic Stress Disorder: DSM-IV and Beyond. Edited by Davidson JRT, Foa EB. Washington, DC, American Psychiatric Press (in press)

Kilpatrick DG, Veronen LJ, Best CL: Factors predicting psychological distress among rape victims, in Trauma and Its Wake. Edited by Figley CR. New York, Brunner/Mazel, 1985a, pp 113–141

Kilpatrick DG, Best CL, Veronen LJ, et al: Mental health correlates of criminal victimization: a random community survey. J Consult Clin Psychol 53:866–873, 1985b

Kilpatrick DG, Saunders BE, Veronen LJ, et al: Criminal victimization: lifetime prevalence, reporting to police, and psychological impact. Crime and Delinquency 33:479–489, 1987a

Kilpatrick DG, Veronen LJ, Saunders BE, et al: The psychological impact of crime: a study of randomly surveyed crime victims (Final Report, Grant No 84-IJ-CX-0039). Washington, DC, National Institute of Justice, 1987b

Kilpatrick DG, Saunders BE, Amick-McMullan A, et al: Victim and crime factors associated with the development of crime-related post-traumatic stress disorder. Behavior Therapy 20:199–214, 1989

Lazarus RS, Folkman S: Stress, Appraisal, and Coping. New York, Springer, 1984

Lindy JD, Grace M: The recovery environment: continuing stressor versus a healing psychosocial space, in Disasters and Mental Health: Contemporary Perspectives and Innovations in Services to Disaster Victims. Edited by

Sowder BJ, Lystad M. Washington, DC, American Psychiatric Press, 1986, pp 137–149

Madakasira S, O'Brien KF: Acute posttraumatic stress disorder in victims of natural disaster. J Nerv Ment Dis 175:286–290, 1987

Maida CA, Gordon NS, Steinberg A, et al: Psychosocial impact of disasters: victims of the Baldwin Hills fire. Journal of Traumatic Stress 2:37–48, 1989

Maslow AH: Toward a Psychology of Being. New York, Van Nostrand Reinhold, 1968

Meichenbaum D: Stress Inoculation Training. Elmsford, NY, Pergamon, 1985

Mitchell J, Bray G: Emergency Services Stress: Guidelines for Preserving the Health and Careers of Emergency Services Personnel. Englewood Cliffs, NJ, Prentice-Hall, 1990

Shaw D, Freedy J, Jarrell P, et al: The relationship between loss of resources and clinical symptomatology among survivors of a natural disaster: a clinical application of the Conservation of Resources model. Poster presented at the 24th annual meeting of the Association for the Advancement of Behavior Therapy, San Francisco, CA, November 1990

Shore JH, Tatum E, Vollmer WM: Evaluation of mental health effects of disaster: Mount St. Helen's eruption. Am J Public Health 76:76–83, 1986

Solomon SD: Research issues in assessing disaster's effects, in Psychosocial Aspects of Disaster. Edited by Gist R, Lubin B. New York, Wiley, 1989, pp 308–340

Solomon SD, Canino G: The appropriateness of DSM-III-R criteria for posttraumatic stress disorder. Compr Psychiatry 31:227–237, 1990

Spielberger CD: Manual for the State-Trait Anxiety Inventory, Revised Edition. Palo Alto, CA, Consulting Psychologists Press, 1983

Stack CB: All Our Kin: Strategies for Survival in a Black Community. New York, Harper & Row, 1974

Veronen LJ, Kilpatrick DG: Stress management for rape victims, in Stress Reduction and Prevention. Edited by Meichenbaum D, Jaremko M. New York, Plenum, 1983, pp 341–374

Wortman CB, Silver RC: Coping with irrevocable loss, in Cataclysms, Crises, and Catastrophes: Psychology in Action. Edited by VandenBos GR, Bryant BK. Washington, DC, American Psychological Association, 1987, pp 189–235

Chapter 2

Nature and Treatment of Acute Stress Reactions

Peter Forster, M.D.

*I*n a turbulent world, the recognition and appropriate treatment of the psychological consequences of traumatic stress are urgent health needs. By one estimate, 1% of the American population suffers from post-traumatic stress disorder (PTSD) (Helzer et al. 1987). This estimate does not include the largest group of individuals who experience these symptoms of stress response: those whose symptoms are at least partly resolved during the first few weeks after exposure to trauma.

Sources of Traumatic Stress

It is worth reviewing some of the many sources of traumatic stress before discussing the natural course of traumatic stress response and its appropriate treatment. Acute stress response symptoms have been identified in both child and adult victims of urban violence (Davis and Friedman 1985; Peterson 1986; Pynoos et al. 1987), including victims of rape (Dahl 1989; DiVasto 1985; Libow and Doty 1979; Mezey and Taylor 1988; Rose 1986) and domestic violence (Kemp et al. 1991). A recent study of an urban population documented that of those people exposed to violence, 23% developed PTSD (Breslau et al. 1991). Of all Americans, 8% die unexpectedly as a result of accidents, suicide, or murder (Rynearson 1986), leaving behind as secondary victims relatives and friends who will experience the intrusive and avoidant symptoms of traumatic bereavement (Cella et al. 1988; Horowitz 1986; Raphael 1977; Rynearson 1986; Sheskin and Wallace 1976; Taylor 1987).

Reports from around the world document similar patterns of acute stress response symptoms among the victims of earthquakes (Gavalya

1987; Lima et al. 1989), floods (Phifer et al. 1988), cyclones or tornadoes (Madakasira and O'Brien 1987; Parker 1975), and volcanoes
(Shore et al. 1986). Disasters caused by humans produce similar symptoms. In one of the first studies of civilian victims of traumatic stress,
Lindemann (1944) reported acute stress response symptoms in almost
all of the victims of the November 1942 Coconut Grove nightclub fire
in Boston, Massachusetts. These findings have been confirmed and
elaborated on in several more recent studies (Gleser et al. 1981;
Weisaeth 1989b).

Several groups have been identified as being at particularly high
risk of developing acute and chronic stress response symptoms. Despite
an ethic of toughness in adversity, symptoms are common among fire
fighters (Hytten and Hasle 1989; McFarlane 1988b), police officers
(Duckworth 1986), and other medical and rescue personnel (Durham et
al. 1985; Jones 1985; Raphael et al. 1983). Acute and chronic stress
response symptoms are common in combat soldiers experiencing heavy
combat (Grinker and Seigel 1963; Rahe 1988; Silverman 1986; Spiegel
et al. 1988). Indeed, much of our knowledge about the symptoms of
stress responses is based on descriptions of "battle shock," "battle
fatigue," or "combat stress reactions" in the American veterans of
recent wars.

Many recent immigrants to the United States are refugees from
terrorism, torture, and state-sponsored violence and oppression and
suffer the acute and chronic manifestations of stress response (Goldfeld
et al. 1988; Simon and Blum 1987). These severely traumatized individuals are difficult to help because their terrible suffering makes them
fear contact with perceived authority figures.

America's urban poor are exposed to shocking levels of violence,
crime, and homicide outside their homes. One in seven young black
men will die from homicide or suicide. Many children and adolescents,
growing up in the most impoverished neighborhoods in American
cities, have been exposed to repeated violence and death in their homes,
schools, and communities.

Course of Acute Reactions

As this brief survey demonstrates, sources of traumatic stress in our
lives are many and varied. Because of this diversity, the nature of acute
stress reactions varies to some extent from individual to individual and

from one stressor to another. However, there are certain common patterns. The initial, transient reaction is one of outcry and alarm. The fear and arousal during this first *outcry* part of the *response phase* usually last only a few minutes. The outcry is often brief, because there is generally an urgent need for a response to a traumatic event.

The second half of the response phase consists of *repair and early recovery*. Where there is such a need for action, most individuals are effective at mobilizing themselves to provide support and help, organizing their efforts in adaptive and innovative ways (Burgess 1985; Duffy 1988; Tierney 1989). A very small number of traumatized individuals demonstrate severe impairment because of fear and act irrationally. Another very small number of individuals are overwhelmed by the traumatic event and are unable to act at all. A larger number of individuals, perhaps one-quarter to one-third, show little response, or an extremely calm and rational response, to the trauma and seem to function even more effectively than they did before the event. Most individuals fall between these extremes, generally being able to do what needs to be done during the repair and early recovery phase, but at times experiencing symptoms of autonomic nervous system arousal, fear, anxiety, outrage, anger, disbelief, denial, or brief periods of psychomotor retardation and emotional withdrawal.

These patterns of response may be affected by the context of the traumatic event. Symptoms of shock, immobilization, withdrawal, and avoidance are more common in those people who are helpless to act, when no response is possible or helpful. Those who are exposed to severe or repetitive traumatic stress may have more symptoms of autonomic nervous system arousal, including tics and adventitious body movements. Stress reactions to single events are primarily manifested by symptoms of anxiety and arousal during the response phase, and reactions to multiple or chronic psychiatric trauma often are manifested by symptoms of exhaustion or depression (Rahe 1988).

Following the full response phase, which may last hours to days, there is usually an *adaptation phase,* which is marked by alternating states of denial and intrusion. Occasionally, the adaptation phase may be delayed (McFarlane 1988a), especially when the work of recovery, reconstruction, or self-preservation is all-consuming (McFarlane and Raphael 1984). During the adaptation phase, reminders and images of the traumatic event intrude into daily life in disturbing ways. Intrusive symptoms may include hypervigilance, easy startle, insomnia, nightmares, and intrusive thoughts, emotions, or behaviors (Horowitz 1986). Perhaps as a response to these intrusive symptoms, denial and avoidance also play a large role in the experience of individuals in the adaptation phase. Symptoms of denial include decreased attention, partial amnesia about the event, decreased emotional awareness, avoidance of intimate contact with others, a decreased ability to process information and think creatively, and a decreased willingness to talk about or think about the traumatic event. Intrusive symptoms usually subside during the first part of the adaptation phase. Often the last intrusive symptoms to resolve are fearful nightmares, and these are usually gone within 4–6 weeks.

During the latter half of the adaptation phase, denial and avoidance become more prominent. Traumatized individuals often begin to mobilize more effective coping responses, but their affect may become dramatically more negative and hostile. There may be a marked decrease in frustration tolerance, an increase in complaining, a noticeable loss of humor, and in some cases a period of nearly paranoid mistrust of the efforts of others. This can be particularly problematic for those who are trying to help victims of trauma, who are often viewed with extreme suspicion (Cranshaw 1963; Sokol 1989; Wilkinson 1983). It can also make it difficult for others who may have been traumatized and are struggling to understand and adapt to their emotional experiences: they may find themselves without anyone to talk to.

During this last part of the adaptation phase there is often a marked increase in somatic anxiety symptoms, including headaches, nausea, diarrhea, vomiting, muscle aches, restlessness, dizziness, tremor, sweating, and general fatigue (Dahl 1989; Feinstein 1989; Gleser et al. 1981). During this phase, weeks to months after the traumatic event, there can be a dramatic increase in visits to physicians and in psychosomatic illnesses (Adams and Adams 1984).

Although the type of symptoms and a very rough sense of the normal time course of response to trauma usually remain the same from traumatic event to traumatic event, events can differ substantially in terms of the severity and duration of symptoms, depending on the nature of the trauma. This variation, combined with a remarkable heterogeneity in study methods, has lead to a lack of consensus in the literature about when an adjustment reaction, which is expected to resolve, becomes a chronic stress reaction (M. A. Green and Berlin 1987). According to DSM-III-R (American Psychiatric Association

1987), 1 month is the criterion for the diagnosis of ṖTSD. A number of studies suggest that a more appropriate point for distinguishing between acute adjustment reactions and chronic stress reactions is 3–4 months. This was the experience of clinicians working with victims of the October 1989 earthquake in San Francisco, and also the experience of clinicians working with victims of a cyclone (Fairley et al. 1986), with victims of sexual assault (Atkeson et al. 1982), victims of bombardment in Lebanon (Saigh 1988), and victims of an oil rig disaster in the North Sea (Holen 1991). Among the last symptoms to resolve are disturbing dreams, somatic anxiety, and illness visits to physicians, but these usually have decreased dramatically by the third or fourth month. Most of those with significant stress response symptoms that persist beyond 3–4 months are likely to experience chronic or intermittent symptoms lasting for months or years.

Reactions Among Children

Considerable attention has been paid to the reactions of children to traumatic stress, at least in part because children may need special attention to prevent chronic symptoms of PTSD (Kinzie et al. 1989; Terr 1981, 1983a, 1988). All of the typical symptoms of stress response reactions have been documented in children following acute traumatic exposure (A. H. Green 1983; Pynoos et al. 1987), although symptoms may vary somewhat from the normal patterns seen in adults, depending on the maturational level of the child.

Some studies have noted that impairment in social function is less prominent in children than in adults (Gleser et al. 1981); other studies suggest that adults may not be aware of the full impact of traumatic stress on children without careful questioning (Terr 1983b; Yule et al. 1990). For instance, parents may not appreciate the full extent of the trauma's effects because behavior at school is often more severely affected than behavior at home (McFarlane 1987a).

Most children, especially younger children, develop a strong fear of being alone and display behavior that may be perceived as over-dependence (Bloch et al. 1956). Powerful phobias that can generalize and develop an almost supernatural quality are not uncommon (Bloch et al. 1956; Dollinger et al. 1984; Kinzie et al. 1989; Stoddard et al. 1989; Terr 1983b), as are severe nightmares or night terrors (Bloch et al. 1956) and regression to a previous level of function, including enuresis in younger children (Stoddard et al. 1989).

Magical beliefs are prominent in younger children (Brett et al. 1988), along with misperceptions of the duration of time and sequences of events (Terr 1983b). Other common symptoms seen in children include foreshortened sense of the future; somatization (Brett et al. 1988; Terr 1983b); aggressive play, which may obsessively repeat or reenact the trauma, particularly in children exposed to child abuse (Bloch et al. 1956; A. H. Green 1983; Terr 1983b); confusion about the meaning of death; and worry about parental reactions (Terr 1983b). This quick review of traumatic stress reactions highlights some of the special needs for the care of children, but it also points out the need for much clearer answers to questions about course, outcome, and prognosis in this vulnerable population.

Psychobiology of Stress Reactions

The similarity of symptoms across many different types of traumatic stressors suggests a common biological substrate for stress response syndromes and PTSD. Stress responses appear to be mediated, at least in part, by alterations in catecholamine systems and by the release of adrenocortical hormones and hypothalamic and pituitary-releasing factors (Glavin 1985; Silverman 1986; van der Kolk et al. 1985; Ziegler et al. 1985). Acutely, there is an increased release of both catecholamines and cortisol. In chronic reactions, the hypothalamic-pituitary-adrenal (HPA) axis, which is responsible for the release of cortisol, remains stimulated; however, catecholamine levels decrease toward baseline as catecholamine stores are depleted.

Chronic stress reactions appear to be much more common when exposure to stress is uncontrollable (Anisman et al. 1980, 1984; Arthur 1987; Breier 1989; Breier et al. 1987; Haracz et al. 1988; Miller et al. 1970; Rahe 1988; Simson et al. 1986; Weiss and Simson 1988; Weiss et al. 1981, 1982). Animals exposed to uncontrollable stress show reactions that are strikingly similar to "combat fatigue" and the other chronic stress reactions first described in the aftermath of World War I and World War II (Rahe 1988). In humans, several studies point to alterations in the HPA axis (Mason et al. 1986, 1988; M. A. Smith et al. 1990), in catecholamine levels (Mason et al. 1988), and in catecholamine receptor sensitivity (Lerer et al. 1987) in cases of chronic PTSD. There is also at least one report of alterations in catecholamines in acute stress reactions (Baum et al. 1983). These studies highlight the role that depletion of catecholamines combined with persistently elevated cortisol plays in the development of chronic stress reactions. They emphasize the link between these profound neurochemical changes and the apparent helplessness of the victim (Anisman et al. 1984; Rahe 1988; Weiss and Simson 1988; Weiss et al. 1981, 1982). Suggestive studies show that pretreatment with a monoamine oxidase inhibitor or a tricyclic antidepressant prevents stress-induced "behavioral depression" (Simson et al. 1986). Thus, biochemical studies may lead to new and powerful techniques for assaying and treating stress reactions.

Animal and human data also point to alterations in pain sensitivity and endorphin levels in individuals with acute and chronic stress reactions (Hoffman et al. 1989; Maier and Keith 1987; Troullos et al. 1989). A typical stress response syndrome may be accompanied by relative analgesia. Perhaps this explains the self-destructive reexposure to traumatic events seen in some victims of trauma.

A common source for many of the alterations in neuroendocrine systems may be the formation of "traumatic memories" (McGee 1984; Pitman 1989; R. L. Solomon and Wynne 1954). These particularly vivid memories, which are laid down at a time of high arousal, in the presence of high levels of corticosteroids and catecholamines, seem to be less vulnerable to extinction and more likely to intrude into everyday life than ordinary memories. These memories also tend to be more vivid and less complex than ordinary memory: easier to reexperience than to describe or explain. An important approach to the treatment of acute stress reactions, and one that is shared by many psychotherapies, focuses on the importance of integrating and reencoding these traumatic memories as verbal memories—either by discussing them in therapy or by describing them in a written journal.

Risk Factors

The variability in responses to traumatic stress among different individuals experiencing different traumatic events has led to a search for risk factors for the most severe acute stress reactions. The largest risk factor is the intensity of the traumatic stress (Durham et al. 1985; Gleser et al. 1981; Shore et al. 1986; Silverman 1986; Weisaeth 1989a). The severity of a stressor can be rated by outside observers, and these "objective" assessments of the severity of a stressor correlate quite well with the development of stress reactions. However, subjective factors also play a role; feelings of guilt about one's role in the traumatic event are highly related to the development of stress reactions (Catherall 1986; Duckworth 1986; Gleser et al. 1981; Taylor 1987). A sense of helplessness about the event is also a significant risk factor for the development of a traumatic stress reaction and is an important subjective factor in assessing the intensity of the traumatic stressor (Raphael et al. 1983).

There is a broad consensus about the critical role of social support in mediating acute stress reactions (Beiser et al. 1989; Bromet et al. 1982; Cook and Bickman 1990; Durham et al. 1985; Evans 1978; Gleser et al. 1981; Libow and Doty 1979; Madakasira and O'Brien 1987; van der Kolk 1987), although at the highest levels of traumatic stress the effect of community support may be less important (Boulanger 1986). Those victims with strong levels of social support have the fewest symptoms and the shortest duration of an acute stress response. Communities that draw together in a time of crisis have fewer individuals with stress response symptoms, and those groups that typically have low levels of support experience the most severe stress symptoms. Tragically, social support may disappear as a consequence of disasters. Our need for a sense of a "just" world may lead us to blame the victim for the misfortune (Gleser et al. 1981; Libow and Doty 1979). Similarly, so that we do not feel vulnerable to traumatic events ourselves, we may defensively attribute the victim's misfortunes to some intrinsic characteristic that distinguishes the victim from ourselves.

For most individuals exposed to traumatic stress, social support buffers against traumatic stress by helping the individuals to find a "meaning" for the event (Catherall 1986; Solkoff et al. 1986) and to rediscover hope. However, "social support" that does not permit a discussion of reactions to the stressful event may be worse than no support at all (Z. Solomon et al. 1987a). My own experience following the San Francisco earthquake was that caregivers often experienced the highest levels of stress because they were prevented from sharing their feelings by the need to shelter and care for their dependents. Similar findings followed the events in Pennsylvania at Three Mile Island in March 1979 and the flood at Buffalo Creek, West Virginia, in February 1972: those with children were most affected by the uncertainty (Bromet et al. 1982; Gleser et al. 1981).

Several studies note that multiple concurrent stressors may be more severe than a single stressor of similar intensity (Baum et al.

1983; Cowan and Murphy 1985; McFarlane 1988a). The most severe traumatic stress reactions almost always happen in the presence of multiple concurrent stressors. Unfortunately, in our increasingly urban world, we are all at increasing risk for stress reactions, since traumatic stress that occurs in high-density areas may be particularly troublesome (Fleming et al. 1987).

Pretraumatic risk factors for acute stress reactions include prior losses or traumas, especially childhood and adolescent losses (van der Kolk 1987). After the San Francisco earthquake, one of the groups most profoundly affected by the traumatic event were Southeast Asian refugees who had recently fled from the trauma of war. Many of them left their community, homes, and jobs in San Francisco to flee to safer central California locations.

The question of whether predisaster psychopathology predicts postdisaster coping remains controversial. Several studies identified anxiety or affective illness as a significant risk factor (Hendin and Haas 1984; North et al. 1989; Silverman 1986). E. M. Smith et al. (1990) reported that people with pretraumatic risk factors may experience stress response symptoms after relatively low exposures to new traumatic events and need to have interventions specifically targeted toward them. However, Gibbs (1989) was unable to confirm this finding.

Others at high risk include the very young (Silverman 1986; Terr 1983a) and the very old (Gleser et al. 1981), although there is controversy about the risk for older children and adolescents (Gleser et al. 1981). Women appear to be at greater risk than men (Erikson 1976; Gleser et al. 1981), and people with more education appear to be at lower risk (Gleser et al. 1981).

Preexisting adaptive or maladaptive coping styles can have a profound impact on physiological and psychological responses to acute stress (Vickers 1988). Avoidance of reminders of the traumatic event can be adaptive in the immediate aftermath of trauma (Bourne et al. 1967; Durham et al. 1985). In one study, avoidance was associated with a short-term decrease in symptoms of depression (Beiser et al. 1989). Intellectualization—the notion that "it could be worse"—may be an especially helpful form of distancing in those working with the victims of trauma (Durham et al. 1985). However, persistent avoidance or denial can be severely detrimental, particularly if it prevents the victim from getting help and from receiving social support (Binder 1981; McFarlane 1988a, 1988b; Z. Solomon 1989) or if it leads to phobic limitations on activities of daily life (Keane et al. 1985a, 1985b; Lyons and Keane 1989). Long-term denial is not useful. Over time, avoiding memories can lead to a decrease in social interaction and intimacy and a marked increase in illness behavior, psychosomatic symptoms, and psychological stress. In a study of Israeli veterans, reality-based coping styles were clearly preferable to avoidance, in terms of long-term psychiatric outcome (Z. Solomon et al. 1991). Confronting traumas has been associated with reductions in physiological activation and an improvement in psychosomatic stress symptoms and illness rates in several studies (Pennebaker et al. 1987, 1988). Implosion therapy of PTSD is just one useful therapy that is based on the observation that exposing oneself to traumatic, walled-off memories of the event is therapeutic.

Intervention for Acute Traumatic Stress

The best intervention for potential victims of traumatic stress is prevention. Psychiatrists and other mental health professionals can appropriately speak about the impact of increasing levels of violence in our world. Although natural disasters cannot be prevented, they can be prepared for. These preparations should include plans for coping with the psychological responses to traumatic stress.

In the immediate aftermath of a traumatic event, survivors need to receive reassurance that they are safe; they need to be given help mastering their acute anxiety; and they need to be given an opportunity to share their story at least once or twice (Rahe 1988). Taking care of the injured and providing shelter and support will obviously have highest priority, but even within the first few minutes to hours after a disaster, consideration needs to be given to the appropriate use of radio, television, and newspapers to distribute essential information, to encourage a calm and pragmatic response to the trauma, and to instill tempered optimism. Early intervention can be extremely powerful and may help prevent long-term problems (Raphael 1977; Sokol 1989). It has been repeatedly shown that the factors involved in a good outcome from traumatic stress include the development of a sense of cohesion and morale and a belief in the effectiveness of community leadership (Belenky et al. 1985; McCaughey 1985).

After an initial period of up to a week of relatively high morale, disillusionment often sets in a few weeks to a month after a major community disaster. In victims of personal tragedies, this disillusionment may occur much sooner. In either case, skepticism about the motives of help providers can make psychological interventions more difficult (Lindy 1985).

Mental health experts can play a key role by delivering a coherent message about the long-term psychological consequences of a traumatic event. Victims need to hear that a *normal* response to traumatic stress includes symptoms of anxiety, insomnia, and hyperarousal. These symptoms may be followed by a period of mild depressive symptoms, but almost all individuals (perhaps except those severely traumatized) can expect substantial recovery within 1–2 months (Figley 1989; McGee 1984; Z. Solomon and Oppenheimer 1986). "Predicting symptoms" or normalizing the common experiences of victims of traumatic stress can be extremely reassuring and provide the entrée into a traumatized community (Figley 1989). Flashbacks, nightmares, and hyperarousal symptoms may be a normal consequence of the formation of traumatic memories (McGee 1984), and emphasizing the continuity between these experiences and normal life and normal memory can be reassuring.

Victims of traumatic events need to receive strong and explicit encouragement to take care of physical health needs, including diet, exercise, and reestablishing regular sleep patterns. Traumatized individuals should be encouraged to resume as much of their life as possible: relatively rapid resumption of normal activity should be expected. Newspaper articles and pamphlets that describe the symptoms of traumatic stress reactions can be extremely reassuring. Lists of treatment resources, including hot lines and brief supportive groups, should be distributed throughout the community. Victims should be encouraged to write down or share their experiences at least once. Sharing experiences with a sympathetic listener can be extremely helpful. Failing that, writing the most troubling experiences in a journal can be another way of gaining some emotional perspective on the events.

Rebuilding one's sense of competency is essential to full recovery, whether this is through a resumption of physical activity, social contacts, or a return to work (Folkman and Lazarus 1980; Gleser et al. 1981; Rahe 1988). In one report, a pilot's ability to master a crash was dramatically enhanced by his use of simulator training equipment, which allowed him to regain a sense of competency as a pilot (Hytten and Hasle 1989).

Although the media play a vital role in disseminating information, individuals need to avoid overexposing themselves to scenes of the traumatic event (McFarlane 1988a). Especially when a threat of further hazard persists, too much exposure to images of disaster in the media can increase stress reactions (Baum et al. 1983; Bromet et al. 1982). Of course, avoiding overexposure should not extend so far that it prevents necessary preparation and prevention from taking place or leads to physical inactivity, a sense of hopelessness, or isolation from one's community.

Among the most effective interventions following a disaster (or a situation where several individuals are affected by traumatic stress) is the formation of support groups. Because social factors are so important in the outcome of traumatic stress reactions, a group model for brief intervention makes intuitive sense (van der Kolk 1987). A dramatic illustration of this principle was the importance of group cohesion for survival during World War II concentration camps (Eitinger 1964; Klein 1974). Although there are no controlled trials of support groups, they have been widely and successfully used for victims of various different traumatic events, including victims of rape (Yassen and Glass 1984), battered women, and war veterans (Walker and Nash 1981; van der Kolk 1987). A group intervention may be especially helpful for families and children (Yule et al. 1990).

A one- or two-session group debriefing has been widely described as a formal way of reviewing events and understanding them, as well as a way of educating victims about the possible psychological consequences of traumatic stress (Dunning 1988; Mitchell 1984). In many circumstances (particularly involving professionals and work groups), this model has been very effective. Its structure, its emphasis on support and information, and the fact that it includes all victims, regardless of individual willingness to acknowledge the need for social or psychological support, prevent individuals from feeling too psychologically vulnerable or burdened by participating in the groups.

Brief individual treatment can also be extremely effective. Short-term therapy (often less than 12 sessions) may be preferable to long-term therapy because of the risk that the victim may develop a dependence on external support in longer-term therapy (Deitz 1986; Horowitz 1976; Marmar and Horowitz 1988; van der Kolk 1987). The goal of short-term therapies is to work through and review unassimilated thoughts and feelings in a way that allows the individual to understand the significance of the event without feeling vulnerable or demoralized.

Affected families are often extremely distressed as the result of traumatic experiences. Caregivers may struggle to deal with their own responses to traumatic stress while providing support to those who depend on them. Brief family therapy that clarifies roles and expectations can be very helpful and can give families a much-needed vocabulary for talking about their needs and experiences (Figley 1989; Harris 1991; Tierney 1989).

Treatment of Children

Early intervention is particularly important for children (Terr 1983b). The first step is teaching parents about the nature of traumatic stress reactions. Otherwise, family members may misinterpret the responses of children to traumatic events and misdirect their efforts to help children cope with the traumatic event. Traumatized families are frequently characterized by increased conflict, irritability, and withdrawal. Instilling hope and normalizing the acute stress response symptoms can strengthen family ties (Figley 1989; McFarlane 1987a). Caregivers may need permission to take care of their own needs before attempting to satisfy the needs for support and reassurance from others. If not, they may inadvertently convey a sense of being overwhelmed or unsupportive to those they are trying to comfort (Bloch et al. 1956). Studies of fire victims in Australia (McFarlane 1987a, 1987b) and of tornado victims in the Midwest (Bloch et al. 1956) showed that the adjustment of parents was a very important determinant of the adjustment of children to a traumatic event. Although it would be ideal if caregivers could always be calm, supportive, and well-adjusted, achieving this state takes careful attention to personal needs for support of reassurance.

Parents should tolerate a brief period of regression and encourage children to express their feelings, teaching in part by example (Terr 1983b). Children have a strong need for dependability after a frightening traumatic event. Special care should be paid to maintaining normal daily routines and fostering the return of a sense of security and confidence. To avoid a contagion of fear, reexposure via television and radio should be limited. Trauma-related play should be supervised to prevent an obsessive repetition of traumatic themes without any resolution of fears (Terr 1983b). Play therapy that does work through the traumatic fears can be helpful (Heimlich 1987), especially if it leads to new and more positive endings to traumatic play (Terr 1983b). In addition to play therapy, there is one case report that points to the use of flooding (Saigh 1986) and two reports of the effective use of group psychotherapy in children (Terr 1983b; Yule et al. 1990). Three authors have suggested that longer-term therapy may be necessary for many trauma-exposed children (Burke et al. 1986; Dreman and Cohen 1990; Terr 1983b). In a disaster, this may be difficult to arrange. The lack of long-term resources should not prevent timely crisis intervention.

Appropriate Pharmacotherapy of Stress Reactions

In traumatized adults, if symptoms persist or are particularly severe despite the provision of information and support, short-term pharmacotherapy may be indicated. Benzodiazepines have been shown to reverse many of the neurochemical alterations produced by stress (Segal 1981; Torrellas et al. 1980; Ziegler et al. 1984). Sleep deprivation can have a profound impact on physical and psychological health (Evans 1978; Rechtschaffen et al. 1989), and early relief from stress response symptoms can be indefinitely delayed by the severe insomnia that is often a consequence of trauma.

Factors that are particularly likely to be responsive to short-term treatment with benzodiazepines include intrusive daytime memories, troubled sleep, and nightmares. Troubled sleep is common and is often the most persistent symptom of an acute stress reaction; up to 70% of individuals experience a serious sleep disturbance (Astrom et al. 1989; Hefez et al. 1987). Human and animal studies have demonstrated the profound impact of significant sleep deprivation on psychological, physiological, and neuroendocrine measures of stress (Bergmann et al. 1989; Everson et al. 1989; Gonzalez-Santos et al. 1989; Horne 1986; Meyerhoff et al. 1988; Nishihara and Mori 1988; Rechtschaffen et al. 1989; Shouse 1988; Zwicker and Calil 1986). Most of these effects are readily reversible by sleep, particularly slow-wave sleep (Everson et al. 1989; Horne 1986). Benzodiazepines appear to be especially effective in treating the insomnia that is related to hyperarousal (Haefley et al. 1983). Nightmares are a common symptom of acute stress reactions (Cernovsky 1988), and benzodiazepines are effective at suppressing rapid eye movement sleep and dreams. It has even been suggested that careful use of benzodiazepines may decrease the tendency of individuals who have suffered a traumatic event to treat their anxiety through increased alcohol use (Caplan et al. 1984). Unfortunately, although benzodiazepines do suppress rapid eye movement sleep and reduce sleep latencies, they may suppress slow-wave sleep and therefore their longer-term use may be counterproductive.

When considering the use of benzodiazepines, clinicians should assess relative contraindications, such as previous benzodiazepine abuse, a history of alcohol or drug abuse (Senay 1989), and perhaps a tendency toward dependent or cluster B personality traits. Benzodiazepines appear to be particularly effective for use in sleep disturbances that last less than 4–5 weeks (Rickels et al. 1985). There have been no reports of benzodiazepine tolerance developing in that short a period of time (Rickels et al. 1989; Swinson et al. 1987; Uhlenhuth et al. 1988; Woods et al. 1988).

Considerable attention has been paid to the potential adverse interactions between pharmacotherapy and psychotherapy. However, interactions between the two are usually positive and are only rarely negative (Caplan et al. 1984; Marks 1976; Marks et al. 1972). Benzodiazepines may actually decrease functional cognitive impairment caused by high levels of anxiety and thus permit more effective psychotherapy (Desai et al. 1983; Woods et al. 1987).

Other pharmacologic treatments for acute stress reactions have been proposed, including the early use of antidepressants. Evidence indicates that pretreatment with a monoamine oxidase inhibitor or a tricyclic antidepressant may prevent stress-induced behavioral depression in animal models (Simson et al. 1986), and there are a few case reports of patients who had a reduction in acute stress symptoms after being treated with tricyclic antidepressants (Blake 1986). Trazodone, carbamazepine, and clonidine, all sedating medications with effects on sympathetic arousal, may have specific roles early in the treatment of acute stress response symptoms. Additional research is necessary to define the appropriate use of these medications in treating acute stress symptoms.

When Do Chronic Reactions Develop?

There has been controversy about how to distinguish between acute and chronic stress reactions. There is probably some case-to-case variation, depending on the nature of the traumatic stress and on the individual who suffers the trauma. DSM-III-R defines PTSD as the persistence of symptoms for more than a month after the traumatic stress (Brett et al. 1988). Recent work suggests that most symptoms can be expected to resolve within 3–4 months. For those whose acute symptoms last longer than 3–4 months, the outcome may depend on treatment efforts as well as on the nature of the traumatic event, and those with symptoms persisting for more than 1 year after a traumatic event are likely to develop a chronic course (Atkeson et al. 1982; Holen 1991; McFarlane 1988a; Murphy 1989). Many who experience symptoms that last 3–4 months, and almost all with symptom duration of 1 year or more, will reexperience these symptoms after reexposure to stress or seasonal reminders. The recurrence of symptoms with stress, or with seasonal reminders, does not necessarily imply the same kind of chronic disability or chronic symptom course as the persistent symptoms seen in the most seriously traumatized individuals (Phifer et al. 1988).

Risk factors for the development of chronic stress reactions (PTSD) are similar to the risk factors for severe acute stress reactions. The severity of early symptoms is a very important warning (Z. Solomon et al. 1987b). The nature of the traumatic experience is another important risk factor, especially if the traumatic event evoked guilt in the traumatized individual or involved deliberate violence or torture (Taylor 1987). The lack of social support, the presence of preexisting trauma, and the presence of preexisting psychiatric problems all predict the development of chronic stress reactions (Catherall 1986; McFarlane 1988a; Murphy 1989; Z. Solomon et al. 1988). Finally, the development of chronic stress reactions may depend more on the duration of the stress than on its intensity. This has been noted particularly in the case of chronic combat stress reactions (Rahe 1988). The distinction between acute and chronic conditions is important because, in contrast to acute stress reactions, the treatment of chronic stress reactions tends to be more long term and is often complicated by comorbid alcohol and drug abuse, as well as financial and legal issues (Leopold and Dillon 1963; Silverman 1986).

Conclusion

Acute stress reactions are important psychiatric problems because there are so many sources of traumatic stress and because prevention and early intervention can eliminate the risk of developing chronic disabling symptoms (Raphael and Middleton 1987; Solkoff et al. 1986). It is common in the aftermath of a traumatic event to minimize the importance of psychological symptoms and to focus on physical disability and physical illness. Early on, this may make sense; however, the denial of the importance of these symptoms by the public, and at times by mental health professionals, can lead to inadequate intervention (Raphael and Middleton 1987). Early posttraumatic experiences are critical to long-term outcome (Solkoff et al. 1986). The impact of chronic stress reactions on physical health, marriage and family relationships, job performance, and social support and friends, as well as on the development of chronic depressive and intrusive symptoms, can be profound. Ignoring the need for intervention is particularly tragic because these acute stress reactions respond so well to limited treatment and interventions.

We have much to learn about the nature and course of acute stress reactions. Research is often difficult to perform in the aftermath of a traumatic event. It can seem irrelevant or disrespectful of the tragedy that faces the victims of traumatic stress. However, future victims will benefit immensely from better knowledge and more effective treatment. To achieve these goals, we need a better understanding of the psychobiology of stress responses, as well as new pharmacologic, psychotherapeutic, and public health strategies for treatment and short-term intervention. As mental health professionals, each of us should take the first step by developing community plans for dealing with traumatic stress and disasters.

References

Adams PR, Adams GR: Mt. St. Helen's ashfall: evidence for a disaster stress reaction. Am Psychol 3:252–260, 1984

American Psychiatric Association: Diagnostic and Statistical Manual of Mental Disorders, 3rd Edition, Revised. Washington, DC, American Psychiatric Association, 1987

Anisman H, Pizzino A, Sklar LS: Coping with stress, norepinephrine depletion and escape performance. Brain Res 191:583–588, 1980

Anisman H, Beauchamp C, Zacharko RM: Effects of inescapable shock and norepinephrine depletion induced by DPS4 on escape performance. Psychopharmacology 83:56–61, 1984

Arthur AZ: Stress as a state of anticipatory vigilance. Percept Mot Skills 64:75–85, 1987

Astrom C, Lunde I, Ortmann J, et al: Sleep disturbances in torture survivors. Acta Neurol Scand 79:150–154, 1989

Atkeson BM, Calhoun M, Karen S, et al: Victims of rape: repeated assessment of depressive symptoms. J Consult Clin Psychol 50:96–102, 1982

Baum A, Gatchel RJ, Schaeffer MA: Emotional, behavioral, and physiological effects of chronic stress at Three Mile Island. J Consult Clin Psychol 51:565–572, 1983

Beiser M, Turner RJ, Ganesan S: Catastrophic stress and factors affecting its consequences among Southeast Asian refugees. Soc Sci Med 28:183–195, 1989

Belenky GL, Noy S, Solomon Z: Battle stress: the Israeli experience. Military Review 7:29–37, 1985

Bergmann BM, Everson CA, Kushida CA, et al: Sleep deprivation in the rat, V: energy use and meditation. Sleep 12:31–41, 1989

Binder R: Difficulties in follow-up of rape victims. Am J Psychiatry 35:534–541, 1981

Blake DJ: Treatment of acute posttraumatic stress disorder with tricyclic antidepressants. South Med J 79:201–204, 1986

Bloch DA, Silber E, Perry SE: Some factors in the emotional reaction of children to disaster. Paper presented at the 11th annual meeting of the American Psychiatric Association, Atlantic City, NJ, May 9–13, 1956

Boulanger G: Predisposition to post-traumatic stress disorder, in The Vietnam Veteran Redefined: Fact and Fiction. Edited by Boulanger G, Kadushin C. Hillsdale, NJ, Lawrence Erlbaum, 1986, pp 37–50

Bourne PG, Rose RM, Mason JW: Urinary 17-OHCS levels: data on seven helicopter ambulance medics in combat. Arch Gen Psychiatry 17:104–110, 1967

Breier A: Experimental approaches to human stress research: assessment of neurobiological mechanisms of stress in volunteers and psychiatric patients. Biol Psychiatry 26:438–462, 1989

Breier A, Albus M, Pickar D, et al: Controllable and uncontrollable stress in humans: alterations in mood and neuroendocrine and psychophysiological function. Am J Psychiatry 144:1419–1425, 1987

Breslau N, Davis G, Andreski P, et al: Traumatic events and post-traumatic stress disorder in an urban population of young adults. Arch Gen Psychiatry 48:216–222, 1991

Brett EA, Spitzer RL, Williams JB: DSM-III-R criteria for post-traumatic stress disorder. Am J Psychiatry 144:1419–1425, 1988

Bromet E, Schulberg HC, Dunn L: Reactions of psychiatric patients to the Three Mile Island nuclear accident. Arch Gen Psychiatry 39:725–730, 1982

Burgess AW: Rape trauma syndrome: a nursing diagnosis. Occupational Health Nursing 33:405–406, 1985

Burke JD Jr, Moccia P, Borus JF, et al: Emotional distress in fifth-grade children ten months after a natural disaster. J Am Acad Child Adolesc Psychiatry 25:536–541, 1986

Caplan RD, Abbey A, Abramis DJ, et al: Tranquilizer use and well-being: a longitudinal study of social and psychological effects. Ann Arbor, MI, Survey Research Center, University of Michigan, 1984

Catherall DR: The support system and amelioration of PTSD in Vietnam veterans. Psychotherapy 23:472–482, 1986

Cella DF, Perry SW, Kulchycky S, et al: Stress and coping in relatives of burn patients: a longitudinal study. Hosp Community Psychiatry 39:159–166, 1988

Cernovsky Z: Refugees' repetitive nightmares. J Clin Psychol 44:702–707, 1988

Cook JD, Bickman L: Social support and psychological symptomatology following a natural disaster. Journal of Traumatic Stress 3:541–556, 1990

Cowan ME, Murphy SA: Identification of post-disaster bereavement risk predictors. Nurs Res 34:71–75, 1985

Cranshaw R: Reactions to a disaster. Arch Gen Psychiatry 9:157–162, 1963

Dahl S: Acute response to rape a PTSD variant. Acta Psychiatr Scand 80:56–62, 1989

Davis RC, Friedman LN: The emotional aftermath of crime and violence, in Trauma and Its Wake: The Study and Treatment of Post-Traumatic Stress Disorder, Vol 1. Edited by Figley CR. New York, Brunner/Mazel, 1985, pp 90–112

Deitz IJ: Time-limited psychotherapy for post-traumatic stress disorder: the traumatized ego and its self-reparative function. Am J Psychother 40:290–299, 1986

Desai N, Taylor-Davies A, Barnett DB: The effects of diazepam and oxprenolol on short term memory individuals of high and low state anxiety. Br J Clin Pharmacol 15:197–202, 1983

DiVasto P: Measuring the aftermath of rape. J Psychosoc Nurs Ment Health Serv 23:33–35, 1985

Dollinger SJ, O'Donnell JP, Stanley AA: Lightening strike disaster: effects on children's fears and worries. J Consult Clin Psychol 52:1028–1038, 1984

Dreman S, Cohen E: Children of victims of terrorism revisited: integrating individual and family treatment approaches. Am J Orthopsychiatry 60:204–209, 1990

Duckworth DH: Psychological problems arising from disaster work. Stress Medicine 2:315–323, 1986

Duffy JC: The Porter lecture: common psychological themes in societies' reaction to terrorism and disasters. Milit Med 153:387–390, 1988

Dunning C: Intervention strategies for emergency workers, in Mental Health Response to Mass Emergencies: Theory and Practice. Edited by Lystad M. New York, Brunner/Mazel, 1988, pp 284–307

Durham TW, McCammon SL, Allison J: The psychological impact of disaster on rescue personnel. Ann Emerg Med 14:664–668, 1985

Eitinger L: Concentration Camp Survivors in Norway and Israel. Olso, Norway, Universitetsforlaget, 1964

Erikson KT: Disaster at Buffalo Creek: loss of communality at Buffalo Creek. Am J Psychiatry 133:302–305, 1976

Evans HI: Psychotherapy for the rape victim: some treatment models. Hosp Community Psychiatry 2:309–312, 1978

Everson CA, Gilliland MA, Kushida CA, et al: Sleep deprivation in the rat, IX: recovery. Sleep 12:60–67, 1989

Fairley M, Langeluddecke P, Tennant C: Psychological and physical morbidity in the aftermath of a cyclone. Psychol Med 16:671–676, 1986

Feinstein A: Post-traumatic stress disorder: a descriptive study supporting DSM-III-R criteria. Am J Psychiatry 146:665–666, 1989

Figley C: Helping Traumatized Families. San Francisco, CA, Jossey-Bass, 1989

Fleming I, Baum A, Davidson LM, et al: Chronic stress as a factor in physiologic reactivity to challenge. Health Psychol 6:212–237, 1987

Folkman S, Lazarus RS: An analysis of coping in a middle-aged community sample. J Health Soc Behav 21:219–239, 1980

Gavalya AS: Reactions to the Mexican earthquake: case vignettes. Hosp Community Psychiatry 38:1327–1330, 1987

Gibbs MS: Factors in the victim that mediate between disaster and psychopathology: a review. Journal of Traumatic Stress 2:489–514, 1989

Glavin GB: Stress and brain noradrenaline: a review. Neurosci Biobehav Rev 9:233–243, 1985

Gleser GC, Green BL, Winget C: Prolonged Psychosocial Effects of Disaster: A Study of Buffalo Creek. New York, Academic Press, 1981

Goldfeld AE, Mollica RF, Pesavento BH, et al: The physical and psychological sequelae of torture: symptomatology and diagnosis. JAMA 259:2725–2730, 1988

Gonzalez-Santos MR, Gaja-Rodriguez OV, Alonso-Uriarte R, et al: Sleep deprivation and adaptive hormonal responses of healthy men. Arch Androl 22:203–207, 1989

Green AH: Child abuse: dimension of psychological trauma in abused children. J Am Acad Child Psychiatry 22:231–237, 1983

Green MA, Berlin MA: Five psychosocial variables related to the existence of post-traumatic stress disorder symptoms. J Clin Psychol 43:643–649, 1987

Grinker RP, Seigel JP: Men Under Stress. New York, McGraw-Hill, 1963

Haefley W, Polc P, Pieri L, et al: Neuropharmacology of benzodiazepines: synaptic mechanisms and neural basis of action, in The Benzodiazepines: From Molecular Biology to Clinical Practice. Edited by Costa E. New York, Raven, 1983, pp 21–66

Haracz JL, Minor TR, Wilkins JN, et al: Learned helplessness: an experimental model of the DST in rats. Biol Psychiatry 23:388–396, 1988

Harris CJ: A family crisis-intervention model for the treatment of posttraumatic stress reaction. Journal of Traumatic Stress 4(2):195–207, 1991

Hefez A, Metz L, Lavie P: Long-term effects of extreme situational stress on sleep and dreaming. Am J Psychiatry 144:344–347, 1987

Heimlich EP: The use of paraverbal therapy in treating an inaccessible, traumatized child. Am J Psychother 41:299–307, 1987

Helzer JE, Robins LN, McEvoy L: Post-traumatic stress disorder in the general population: findings of the Epidemiologic Catchment Area survey. N Engl J Med 317:1630–1634, 1987

Hendin H, Haas AP: Combat adaption of Vietnam veterans without posttraumatic stress disorders. Am J Psychiatry 141:956–960, 1984

Hoffman L, Burges Watson P, Wilson G, et al: Low plasma beta-endorphin in post-traumatic stress disorder. Aust N Z J Psychiatry 23:269–273, 1989

Holen A: A longitudinal study of the occurrence and persistence of posttraumatic health problems in disaster survivors. Stress Medicine 7:11–17, 1991

Horne JA: Human slow wave sleep. Eur Neurol 25:18–21, 1986

Horowitz MJ: Stress Response Syndromes. New York, Jason Aronson, 1976

Horowitz MJ: Stress-response syndromes: a review of post-traumatic and adjustment disorders. Hosp Community Psychiatry 37:241–249, 1986

Hytten K, Hasle A: Fire fighters: a study of stress and coping. Acta Psychiatr Scand 38:316–322, 1989

Jones DR: Secondary disaster victims: the emotional effects of recovering and identifying human remains. Am J Psychiatry 142:303–307, 1985

Keane TM, Zimering RT, Caddell JM: A behavioral formulation of post-traumatic stress disorder in Vietnam veterans. Behavior Therapist 8:9–12, 1985a

Keane TM, Scott WO, Chavoya GA, et al: Social support in Vietnam veterans with posttraumatic stress disorder: a comparative analysis. J Consult Clin Psychol 53:95–102, 1985b

Kemp A, Rawlings EI, Green BL: Post-traumatic stress disorder (PTSD) in battered women: a shelter sample. Journal of Traumatic Stress 4:137–148, 1991

Kinzie JD, Sack W, Angell R, et al: A three-year follow-up of Cambodian young people traumatized as children. J Am Acad Child Adolesc Psychiatry 28:501–504, 1989

Klein H: Delayed affects and after-effects of severe traumatisation. Israel Annals of Psychiatry and Related Disciplines 12(4):293–303, 1974

Leopold RL, Dillon H: Psycho-anatomy of a disaster: a long-term study of post-traumatic neuroses in survivors of a marine explosion. Am J Psychiatry 119:913–921, 1963

Lerer B, Ebstein RP, Shestatsky M, et al: Cyclic AMP signal transduction in post-traumatic stress disorder. Am J Psychiatry 144:1324–1327, 1987

Libow JA, Doty DW: An exploratory approach to self-blame and self-derogation by rape victims. Am J Orthopsychiatry 49:670–679, 1979

Lima BR, Chavez H, Samaniego N, et al: Disaster severity and emotional disturbance: implications for primary mental health care in developing countries. Acta Psychiatr Scand 79:74–82, 1989

Lindemann E: Symptomatology and management of acute grief. Am J Psychiatry 101:141–148, 1944

Lindy JD: The trauma membrane and other clinical concepts derived from psychotherapeutic work with survivors of natural disasters. Psychiatric Annals 15:153–160, 1985

Lyons J, Keane TM: Implosive therapy for the treatment of combat-related PTSD. Journal of Traumatic Stress 2:137–152, 1989

Madakasira S, O'Brien KF: Acute post-traumatic stress disorder in victims of a natural disaster. J Nerv Ment Dis 175:286–290, 1987

Maier SF, Keith JR: Shock signals and the development of stress-induced analgesia. J Exp Psychol [Anim Behav] 13:226–238, 1987

Marks IM: "Psycholopharmacology": the use of drugs combined with psychological treatment. Proceedings of the Annual Meeting of the American Psychopathological Association 64:108–126, 1976

Marks IM, Viswanathan R, Lipsedge MS, et al: Enhanced relief of phobias by flooding during waning diazepam effect. Br J Psychiatry 121(564):493–505, 1972

Marmar CR, Horowitz MJ: Diagnosis and phase-oriented treatment of post-traumatic stress disorder, in Human Adaptation to Extreme Stress. Edited by Wilson JP, Harel Z, Kahana B. New York, Plenum, 1988, pp 81–103

Mason JW, Giller EL, Kosten TR, et al: Urinary free-cortisol levels in post-traumatic stress disorder patients. J Nerv Ment Dis 174:145–149, 1986

Mason JW, Giller EL, Kosten TR, et al: Elevation of urinary norepinephrine/cortisol ratio in post-traumatic stress disorder. J Nerv Ment Dis 176:498–502, 1988

McCaughey BG: US Coast Guard collision at sea. Journal of Human Stress 11:42–46, 1985

McFarlane AC: Family functioning and overprotection following a natural disaster: the longitudinal effects of post-traumatic morbidity. Aust N Z J Psychiatry 21:210–218, 1987a

McFarlane AC: Post-traumatic phenomena in a longitudinal study of children following a natural disaster. J Am Acad Child Adolesc Psychiatry 26:764–769, 1987b

McFarlane AC: The longitudinal course of post-traumatic morbidity: the range of outcomes and their predictors. J Nerv Ment Dis 176:30–39, 1988a

McFarlane AC: The phenomenology of post-traumatic stress disorder following a natural disaster. J Nerv Ment Dis 176:22–29, 1988b

McFarlane AC, Raphael B: Ash Wednesday: the effects of a fire. Aust N Z J Psychiatry 18:3412–3512, 1984

McGee R: Flashbacks and memory phenomena: a comment on "Flashback Phenomena—Clinical and Diagnostic Dilemmas." J Nerv Ment Dis 172:273–278, 1984

Meyerhoff JL, Oleshansky MA, Mougey EH: Psychological stress increases plasma levels of prolactin, cortisol, and POMC derived peptides in man. Psychosom Med 50:295–303, 1988

Mezey GC, Taylor PJ: Psychological reactions of women who have been raped: a descriptive and comparative study. Br J Psychiatry 152:330–339, 1988

Miller FP, Cox RH Jr, Snodgrass WR, et al: Comparative effects of p-chlorophenylalanine, p-chloroamphetamine and p-chloro-N-methyl-amphetamine on rat brain norepinephrine, serotonin and 5-hydroxy-indole-3-acetic acid. Biochem Pharmacol 19:435–442, 1970

Mitchell JT: Helping the helper, in Role Stressors and Supports for Emergency Workers (DHHS Publ No ADM 85-1908). Edited by Lystad M. Washington, DC, U.S. Government Printing Office, 1984, pp 105–118

Murphy SA: An explanatory model of recovery from disaster loss. Res Nurs Health 12:67–76, 1989

Nishihara K, Mori K: The relationship between waking time and urinary epinephrine in bed-rested humans under conditions involving minimal stress. Int J Psychophysiol 6:133–137, 1988

North CS, Smith EM, McCool RE, et al: Short-term psychopathology in eye-witnesses to mass murder. Hosp Community Psychiatry 40:1293–1295, 1989

Parker G: Psychological disturbance in Darwin evacuees following Cyclone Tracy. Med J Aust 1:650–652, 1975

Pennebaker JW, Hughes CF, O'Heeron RC: The psychophysiology of confession: linking inhibitory and psychosomatic processes. J Pers Soc Psychol 52(4):781–793, 1987

Pennebaker JW, Kiecolt-Glaser JK, Glaser R: Disclosure of traumas and immune function: health implications for psychotherapy. J Consult Clin Psychol 56(2):239–245, 1988

Peterson LG: Acute responses to trauma. Adv Psychosom Med 16:84–92, 1986

Phifer JF, Kaniasty KZ, Norris FH: The impact of natural disaster on the health of older adults: a multiwave prospective study. J Health Soc Behav 29:65–78, 1988

Pitman RK: Post-traumatic stress disorder, hormones, and memory. Biol Psychiatry 26:221–223, 1989

Pynoos RS, Frederick C, Nader K, et al: Life threat and post-traumatic stress in school-age children. Arch Gen Psychiatry 44:1057–1063, 1987

Rahe RH: Acute versus chronic psychological reactions to combat. Milit Med 153:365–372, 1988

Raphael B: Preventative intervention with the recently bereaved. Arch Gen Psychiatry 34:1450–1454, 1977

Raphael B, Middleton W: Mental health responses in a decade of disaster: Australia, 1974–1983. Hosp Community Psychiatry 38:1331–1337, 1987

Raphael B, Singh B, Bradbury L, et al: Who helps the helpers? the effects of disaster on the rescue workers. Omega 124:9–20, 1983

Rechtschaffen A, Bergmann BM, Everson CA, et al: Sleep deprivation in the rat, X: integration and discussion of the findings. Sleep 12:68–87, 1989

Rickels K, Downing RW, Case WG, et al: Six-week trial of diazepam: some clinical observations. J Clin Psychiatry 46:470–474, 1985

Rickels K, Schweizer E, Case WG: Withdrawal problems with anti-anxiety drugs: nature and management, in Psychopharmacology of Anxiety. Edited by Tyrer P. Oxford, Oxford University Press, 1989, pp 283–293

Rose DS: "Worse than death": psychodynamics of rape victims and the need for psychotherapy. Am J Psychiatry 143:817–824, 1986

Rynearson EK: Psychological effects of unnatural dying on bereavement. Psychiatric Annals 16:272–275, 1986

Saigh PA: In vitro flooding in the treatment of a 6-year-old boy's post-traumatic stress disorder. Behav Res Ther 24:685–688, 1986

Saigh PA: Anxiety, depression, and assertion across alternating intervals of stress. J Abnorm Psychol 97:338–341, 1988

Segal M: Effect of diazepam on chronic stress-induced hypertension in the rat. Experientia 37:298–299, 1981

Senay EC: Addictive behaviors and benzodiazepines, 1: abuse liability and physical dependence. Adv Alcohol Subst Abuse 8(1):107–124, 1989

Sheskin A, Wallace SE: Differing bereavements: suicide, natural, and accidental death. Omega 7:229–242, 1976

Shore JH, Tatum EL, Vollmer WM: Psychiatric reactions to disaster: the Mount St. Helens experience. Am J Psychiatry 143:590–595, 1986

Shouse MN: Sleep deprivation increases thalamocortical excitability in the somatomotor pathway, especially during seizure-prone sleep or awakening states in feline seizure models. Exp Neurol 99:664–677, 1988

Silverman JJ: Post-traumatic stress disorder. Adv Psychosom Med 16:115–140, 1986

Simon RI, Blum RA: After the terrorist incident: psychotherapeutic treatment of former hostages. Am J Psychother 41:194–200, 1987

Simson PG, Weiss JM, Ambrose MJ, et al: Infusion of a monoamine oxidase inhibitor into the locus coeruleus can prevent stress-induced behavioral depression. Biol Psychiatry 21:724–734, 1986

Smith EM, North CS, McCool RE, et al: Acute post-disaster psychiatric disorders: identification of persons at risk. Am J Psychiatry 147:194–200, 1990

Smith MA, Davidson J, Ritchie JC, et al: The corticotropin-releasing hormone test in patients with post-traumatic stress disorders: identification of persons at risk. Am J Psychiatry 147:194–200, 1990

Sokol RJ: Early mental health intervention in combat situations: the USS Stark. Milit Med 154:407–409, 1989

Solkoff N, Gray P, Keill S: Which Vietnam veterans develop post-traumatic stress disorders? J Clin Psychiatry 42:687–698, 1986

Solomon RL, Wynne LC: Traumatic avoidance learning: the principles of anxiety conservation and partial irreversibility. Psychol Rev 612:353–385, 1954

Solomon Z: Untreated combat-related PTSD—why some Israeli veterans do not seek help. Isr J Psychiatry Relat Sci 26:111–123, 1989

Solomon Z, Oppenheimer B: Social network variables and stress reaction-lessons from the 1973 Yom-Kippur war. Milit Med 151:12–15, 1986

Solomon Z, Mikulincer M, Freid B, et al: Family characteristic and post traumatic stress disorder: a follow-up of Israeli combat stress reaction casualties. Fam Process 26:383–394, 1987a

Solomon Z, Weisenburg M, Schwarzwald J, et al: Post-traumatic stress disorder among frontline soldiers with combat stress reaction: the 1982 Israeli experience. Am J Psychiatry 144:448–454, 1987b

Solomon Z, Mikulincer M, Avitzur E: Coping, locus of control, social support, and combat-related post-traumatic stress disorder: a prospective study. J Pers Soc Psychol 55:279–285, 1988

Solomon Z, Mikulincer M, Arad R: Monitoring and blunting: implications for combat-related post-traumatic stress disorder. Journal of Traumatic Stress 4(2):209–221, 1991

Spiegel D, Hunt T, Dondershine HE: Dissociation and hypnotizability in post-traumatic stress disorder. Am J Psychiatry 145:301–305, 1988

Stoddard FJ, Norman DK, Murphy JM, et al: Psychiatric outcome of burned children and adolescents. J Am Acad Child Adolesc Psychiatry 28:589–595, 1989

Swinson RP, Pecknold JC, Kirby ME: Benzodiazepine dependence. J Affective Disord 13(2):109–118, 1987

Taylor AJ: A taxonomy of disasters and their victims. J Psychosom Res 31:535–544, 1987

Terr LC: Psychic trauma in children: observations following the Chowchilla school-bus kidnapping. Am J Psychiatry 138:14–19, 1981

Terr LC: Chowchilla revisited: the effects of psychic trauma four years after a school-bus kidnapping. Am J Psychiatry 140:1543–1550, 1983a

Terr LC: Time sense following psychic trauma: a clinical study of ten adults and twenty children. Am J Orthopsychiatry 53:244–261, 1983b

Terr LC: What happens to early memories of trauma? a study of twenty children under age five at the time of documented traumatic events. J Am Acad Child Adolesc Psychiatry 27:96–104, 1988

Tierney KJ: The social and community contexts of disaster, in Psychosocial Aspects of Disaster. Edited by Gist R, Lubin B. New York, Wiley, 1989, pp 11–39

Torrellas A, Guaza C, Borrel J: Effects of acute and prolonged administration of chlordiazepoxide upon the pituitary-adrenal activity and brain catecholamines in sound stressed and unstressed rats. Neurosci Biobehav Rev 5:2289–2295, 1980

Troullos ES, Hargreaves KM, Goldstein DS, et al: Epinephrine suppresses stress-induced increases in plasma immunoreactive beta-endorphin in humans. J Clin Endocrinol Metab 69:546–551, 1989

Uhlenhuth EH, DeWit H, Balter NB, et al: Risks and benefits of long-term benzodiazepine use. J Clin Psychopharmacol 8:161–167, 1988

van der Kolk BA: The role of the group in the origin and resolution of the trauma response, in Psychological Trauma. Edited by van der Kolk BA. Washington, DC, American Psychiatric Press, 1987, pp 153–171

van der Kolk BA, Greenberg M, Boyd H, et al: Inescapable shock, neurotransmitters, and addiction to trauma: toward a psychobiology of post-traumatic stress. Biol Psychiatry 20:314–325, 1985

Vickers RR Jr: Effectiveness of defenses: a significant predictor of cortisol excretion under stress. J Psychosom Res 32:21–29, 1988

Walker JI, Nash JL: Group therapy in the treatment of Vietnam combat veterans. Int J Group Psychother 31:379–389, 1981

Weisaeth L: The stressors and the post-traumatic stress syndrome after an industrial disaster. Acta Psychiatr Scand 80:63–72, 1989a

Weisaeth L: Torture of a Norwegian ship's crew: the torture, stress reactions, and psychiatric after-effects. Acta Psychiatr Scand 80:25–37, 1989b

Weiss JM, Simson PE: Neurochemical and electrophysiological events underlying stress-induced depression in an animal model. Adv Exp Med Biol 245:425–440, 1988

Weiss JM, Goodman PA, Losito BG, et al: Behavioral depression produced by an uncontrollable stressor: relationship to norepinephrine, dopamine, and serotonin levels in various regions of rat brain. Brain Research Review 3:167–205, 1981

Weiss JM, Bailey WH, Goodman PA, et al: A model for neurochemical study of depression, in Behavioral Models and the Analysis of Drug Action. Edited by Spiegelstein MY, Levy A. Amsterdam, Elsevier Scientific, 1982

Wilkinson CB: Aftermath of a disaster: the collapse of the Hyatt-Regency Hotel skywalks. Am J Psychiatry 140:1134–1139, 1983

Woods JH, Katz JL, Winger G: Abuse liability of benzodiazepines. Pharmacol Rev 39:251–413, 1987

Woods JH, Katz JL, Winger G: Use and abuse of benzodiazepines: issues relevant to prescribing. JAMA 260(23):3476–3480, 1988

Yassen J, Glass L: Sexual assault survivor groups. Social Work 37:252–257, 1984

Yule W, Udwin O, Murdoch K: The "Jupiter" sinking: effects on children's fears, depression and anxiety. J Child Psychol Psychiatry 31:1051–1061, 1990

Ziegler G, Ludwig L, Klotz U: Stress protective effects during steady-state conditions of bromazepam. Pharmacopsychiatry 17(6):194–198, 1984

Ziegler MG, Milano AJ, Hull E: The catecholaminergic response to stress and exercise, in The Catecholamines in Psychiatric and Neurologic Disorders. Edited by Lake CR, Ziegler MG. Boston, MA, Butterworth, 1985, pp 37–54

Zwicker A, Calil HM: The effects of REM sleep deprivation on striatal dopamine receptor sites. Pharmacol Biochem Behav 24:809–812, 1986

Chapter 3

Organizing a Disaster Response Program in One's Home Community

Linda S. Austin, M.D.

*T*he purpose of this chapter is to provide a framework for organizing and prioritizing a mental health response to a traumatized community. The scale of such an intervention at first may seem overwhelming to the professional accustomed to responding to individuals or small groups. Fortunately, mass group trauma responds remarkably well to the mass group interventions that may be the treatment of choice for the traumatized community. Traumatized individuals find extraordinary comfort by identification with the community at large and will even shun individual interventions that make them feel as if they are "weaker" than those experiencing similar trauma. The professional's challenge is to stimulate the natural healing processes set into motion by mass group identification by a variety of interventions described in this volume.

An important principle of disaster response is that disasters unfold in a series of stages, determined in part by the nature of the disaster (R. E. Cohen and Ahearn 1980). Different clinical responses are appropriate for different stages of the disaster. For example, children may benefit from group interventions immediately postdisaster, whereas adults may be so preoccupied by responding to physical survival requirements that they may be inaccessible for any mental health interventions for days, weeks, or even months after a disaster (Austin 1991).

My own disaster experience was with Hurricane Hugo in September 1989, which seemed to unfold in slow motion: we had several days of warning before Hugo struck, the hurricane itself lasted for hours, and the recovery extended over months. This is obviously a different sort of time sequence than an earthquake, representing an unpredictable instantaneous disaster, or a war, representing an even more prolonged disaster. Roughly stated, disaster response is composed of four stages: advance planning, the disaster itself, the acute postdisaster period (lasting approximately several weeks), and recovery. In this chapter I address organizational issues of each stage.

Several other general principles overarch the four stages of disaster response. As illustrated in this volume, each disaster is unique, leaving its own particular signature on a particular unique community. The factors that determine the impact of a trauma on a community are detailed by Freedy et al. (Chapter 1, this volume) and R. E. Cohen (Chapter 4, this volume). Quirks of fate have extraordinary significance in determining the outcome of a disaster, such as the day of the week and time an earthquake strikes, or the decision of a mayor whether to order an evacuation for a hurricane. Disaster recovery may also be powerfully affected by events particular to that period, such as the nature and degree of external aid (Raphael 1986). Therefore, although advance planning is always helpful and important, planning must also include the need for great flexibility and sensitivity to the vicissitudes of disaster reactions and recovery and assume that these are inherently unpredictable. The disaster worker is well advised not to make strongly worded predictions of disaster reactions, particularly in public.

Many disaster workers, including many of the authors of this volume, have developed expertise in disaster work not by choice or by training but because of suddenly finding themselves residents of a traumatized community. Formulating a disaster response within one's own community while also restoring one's own life and tending to the emotional needs of self and family is challenging (Raphael and Middleton 1987). Fortunately, there is some parallel between the timing of the psychological needs of a community and the availability of mental health workers to respond. In the acute phases of a disaster, the community members will be preoccupied by meeting their physical needs, just as the mental health workers generally need to care for themselves and their families; a relatively small cadre of workers will be sufficient to respond to acute psychiatric needs within the community. As the recovery progresses, the community will gradually become ready for intervention, just as mental health workers will become gradually ready to provide intervention.

Given that many disaster workers who are residents of a traumatized community may be inexperienced and themselves in a state of emotional upset, consultation with experienced disaster workers in other geographic areas may be extremely useful. Optimally the consultant will be someone with experience in a similar disaster, and caution should be observed not to overgeneralize from the consultant's experience. It would be preferable for the consultant to be of the same discipline as the consultee to provide a shared frame of reference. The consultant may provide important emotional support by "walking" the consultee through the various stages of disaster response and may provide scholarly literature as well as practical information, such as how to contact and negotiate with government agencies and insurance companies. Professional organizations, such as the American Psychiatric Association and the American Psychological Association, have disaster response committees that can provide information and names of appropriate consultants.

Stages of Disaster Response

Planning for a Disaster

The degree and sophistication of disaster planning vary enormously from locality to locality. At the most rudimentary level, state laws generally require regular fire drills in institutions and have certain sites (usually school gymnasiums) designated as emergency shelters. California is an interesting example of a state that has struggled to overcome its own natural denial about the likelihood of a disaster. In many areas of the state, a significant amount of disaster preparedness has taken place; for example, in many school systems all schools must be "quake-proof."

Certain geographic locations are obvious targets for particular forms of disasters. For example, the southeastern coast of the United States predictably is hit by hurricanes of varying intensity every year. In planning for such potential disasters, mental health professionals in general and psychiatrists in particular may make important contributions in several areas. The first is to take an active role in planning for the needs of emergency shelters. Often the high school principal at each shelter site is designated to be in charge of the shelter during a disaster; these principals may have varying degrees of knowledge, training, and enthusiasm for the job. There may be little provision for the medical needs of these local shelters, let alone the mental health needs. This may create obvious problems, especially since homeless mentally ill individuals may take up residence in these shelters until forced out at the "end" of the disaster. Psychiatric disaster preparedness includes collaboration with local officials to staff emergency shelters. Optimally psychiatrists can volunteer to staff shelters during emergencies. It should be remembered, however, that this may result in a given psychiatrist being not only the sole mental health professional at a shelter, but the only medical personnel of any sort whatever. For example, during Hurricane Hugo the "ranking" medical staff person at one shelter was a family practice resident, who delivered a baby and treated diabetic patients at his shelter. Psychiatrists working at disaster sites have reported that during the acute phases of a disaster, general medical skills may be as highly valued as psychiatric skills (Black 1987). Psychiatrists who are uncomfortable with their general medical skills might consider teaming up with another medical colleague at such sites. Medical personnel at a shelter would be well advised to ascertain the provision of basic medical supplies available.

A second important role in the planning stage is to consider arrangements for evacuating psychiatric inpatients. This evacuation may be facilitated by preexisting mutual agreements with a "sister" institution to provide emergency shelter for evacuated patients who cannot be discharged to their homes. In the event of a potential disaster, prudence dictates the evacuation of as many patients as possible to protect their physical safety, to shield them from the enormous anxiety surrounding an anticipated disaster, and to provide them with optimal psychiatric care. At times a facility cannot be fully evacuated; for a discussion of the management of a psychiatric inpatient facility during a disaster, the reader is referred to Arana et al. (Chapter 12, this volume).

When disaster is imminent, it is important to consider mental health personnel resources for the institution or facility for which one is responsible. Mental health care management must decide which personnel are absolutely necessary to provide adequate care for remaining patients and to encourage the evacuation of all other personnel as early as possible. Although it would seem preferable to have a large staff available during a disaster, the challenge of finding food and water for these people in postdisaster conditions may be very difficult. Given the luxury of advanced warning for a disaster, mental health care leadership is well advised to encourage the evacuation of all but a skeleton crew of mental health care workers. There will be abundant opportunities for mental health intervention once safe conditions again prevail.

Several factors are important in the determination of which personnel should stay during a disaster. Family responsibilities may be a determining factor, although in our experience there were so few personnel without families that many staff who remained at the hospital had their children with them. Some personality types may be better suited to working through a disaster than others. During our experiences with Hugo, we noted that personality traits became exaggerated to the point that some individuals became caricatures of themselves: the histrionic became frazzled; the conscientious became heroic; and the unreliable vanished altogether for several days without communication. In planning personnel needs, physical survival needs should not be overlooked: a plumber, cook, or handy person may be as important as a psychiatrist.

During the Disaster

Several studies have described behavior during disaster situations. Quarantelli and Dynes (1973) reported that individuals are able to exhibit situationally adaptive behavior during most disaster situations. Tyhurst (1957) reported that 12%–25% of survivors remain "cool and collected"; 75% appear stunned and bewildered; and 10%–25% become confused or hysterical. Weisaeth (1989) documented that levels of disaster training correlated strongly with adaptive behavior during a disaster and that although the majority of victims displayed diminished cognitive abilities during a disaster, they were able to maintain behavioral control by passively copying the leaders.

These findings corroborate our observations at shelter sites during Hurricane Hugo. Shelter residents were remarkably quiet and responded well to suggestions and soothing from mental health personnel. The psychiatric inpatients were particularly calm; perhaps the disaster experience represented for them an intensification of the passivity inherent in inpatient hospitalization. Shelter residents seemed to benefit from being told in some detail what to expect as they awaited the storm, perhaps representing a form of "on-the-job" training in disaster response. These observations underscore the notion that strong, calm, confident leadership during all phases of disaster activity is required to respond to the regressive nature of the disaster experience.

Acute Postdisaster Stage

Regardless of the nature of the disaster, several concerns require immediate attention after a disaster. The first is to ensure the care of psychiatric inpatients. This includes talking to them about the disaster, attempting to allow them to communicate with their families if it is physically possible, and allowing them to see the nature and extent of the disaster. Staff members who have remained at the inpatient facility during the disaster must be relieved, and work shifts must be established. Further aspects of postdisaster inpatient care are discussed by Arana et al. (Chapter 12, this volume).

A second immediate priority is to develop a system to provide mental health care at the emergency shelters. Typically, even in a predicted disaster, staffing has been arranged hastily to cover just the period of the disaster itself. However, since shelters often must remain open for days or weeks, responsibility for staffing these shelters must be arranged. Although it is not necessary to have a full-time professional at each shelter, "house calls" at shelters may be very useful, as described by Zealberg and Puckett (Chapter 11, this volume).

Many disasters require the immediate assistance of local volunteers, police, fire fighters, or the National Guard. At times the individuals provide aid in extremely harrowing circumstances, such as the workers who freed trapped motorists under the collapsed Nimitz freeway after the San Francisco earthquake in October 1989. These individuals may become quite traumatized by their experiences (Berah et al. 1984; Ersland et al. 1989). The mental health professional may be very helpful by counseling those who are organizing such relief efforts to watch for warning signs that individuals are becoming overwhelmed. The professional may also volunteer to provide large-group "debriefings" (to be described later), to provide mini-marathons (see Terr, Chapter 5, this volume), or to perform individual evaluations for these groups if indicated.

An important priority in the acute postdisaster phase is to develop an intervention program for school-age children as soon as possible. Adults may be able to wait for several weeks to process their feelings about a disaster; children are unable to wait, and teachers will become less motivated to participate if intervention is delayed. Depending on the nature of the disaster, schools may be temporarily closed; however, as soon as the children are back in the class, teachers will need to respond to the children's anxieties in some way. For a relatively local-ized disaster, it may be possible to assign one or more professionals to each school to train teachers in disaster response methods for children. However, if the disaster has affected an entire large community, this may not be feasible. In such a situation, one may, for example, organize a workshop for all principals of the school system to debrief them and teach them classroom intervention techniques, discussed by Terr (Chapter 5, this volume) and Eth (Chapter 6, this volume). It should then become the explicitly stated responsibility of each principal to train his or her teachers in these methods. Depending on the mental health resources of the community, a liaison mental health professional may serve as a consultant to a school or a group of schools. It is important to establish an alliance with school officials, such as the superintendent of schools or the director of school counseling services, to ensure that the principals will respond appropriately.

As soon as it is physically possible, the media will call on mental health professionals to develop stories about the disaster. Often the media will use mental health professionals already known to them, regardless of their level of expertise with disaster response. The orga-nizer of the disaster response should appoint several professionals with experience in media work to serve as spokespersons. Principles of media work are fully discussed by Terr (Chapter 5, this volume) and by Ruben (Chapter 7, this volume). In our experience with Hurricane Hugo, media interviews were the single most effective way to "debrief" the entire population.

Active intervention with the adult population of a community during the acute postdisaster phase depends on conditions that may vary widely according to the disaster. After Hurricane Hugo, we pre-dicted an immediate enormous increase in demand for inpatient and outpatient services. Not only was there no such demand, but for several weeks most of our regular outpatients canceled their appointments to meet their own physical recovery needs. The only calls I received during the first 2 weeks from my regular patients were to inquire if I and my family were physically safe. The inpatient service also did not experience an increased demand for services in the weeks and months after Hugo. Many patients with significant psychiatric illness seemed to put their predisaster symptoms aside temporarily, confirming Rangell's (1976) observation that only when normalcy returns is the luxury of becoming individually neurotic restored.

The community vastly preferred various forms of large (or mass) group therapy, attending such sessions in large numbers. These sessions seemed to allow them to experience all of Charleston, South Carolina, as a healing environment. It should be stressed that this was probably in large part due to the nature of our disaster. We had very few deaths (26 in South Carolina), and the overwhelming loss was property damage (Mayfield 1990). Disasters that produce high death and casualty rates produce different and more severe patterns of symptom formation (Kinston and Rosser 1974) and may well require more individual intervention, as victims struggle to respond to the loss of loved ones or new physical handicaps. However, the need for such individual intervention might not surface for weeks or months, when the shock of the trauma has worn off.

Recovery Phase

The recovery phase may be roughly conceived as beginning several weeks after the recovery. In the case of Hurricane Hugo, recovery issues dominated the community for a solid year after the storm, and the 1-year anniversary was celebrated with parties, observances, and media commentary. Following that, preoccupation with Hugo has lessened considerably. Other disasters, such as the Armenian earthquake in December 1988, which resulted in 25,000 deaths, will have more prolonged recoveries, lasting years or decades.

Many of the activities of the recovery phase are continuations of the acute postdisaster phase. Consultation with schools and rescue groups and interaction with the media continue. However, one of the most important organizational efforts of the recovery phase should be to debrief the population through a variety of large-group techniques. The following theoretical principles should guide mental health workers in responding to traumatized groups, regardless of the site of intervention.

Theoretical considerations in large-group interventions. It may be helpful to conceptualize similarities and differences between individual and group trauma. Both types of events set in motion powerful forces of regression: the sense of smallness, vulnerability, terror, pain, and loss (Black 1987). However, individual trauma may also cause emotional responses that are not necessarily part of mass trauma response, including the sense of shame, isolation, personal blame, and the fear (and perhaps reality) that no one else can truly understand. The "Why me?" question is infinitely more painful than the "Why us?" question because of the echo it contains of personal isolation.

Unlike individualized trauma, mass trauma is potentially subject to the healing forces of group dynamics, which should be thoughtfully and carefully enhanced by the mental health worker. The individual will naturally seek to overcome his or her sense of regressive smallness by identification with the size, power, and courage of the large group, however traumatized it might be. In essence, all of the large-group techniques described in this volume promote the power of group identification by encouraging an open sharing of the traumatic experience within groups.

The history of the Jews is a dramatic example of the power of group identification in responding to group trauma. For several thousand years, Jewish leaders have been able to assist their people through repeated horrific disasters by promoting a sense of affiliation with the large group. Several chapters in this volume illustrate that disaster aid is most successful when it promotes the healing power of a similar sort of group identification, such as that described after the Armenian earthquake in December 1988 and the Guadalupe River drownings in July 1987. By contrast, the healing process in response to a disaster such as Hurricane Hugo in the Virgin Islands (Black, Chapter 10, this volume) may be far more difficult because of the ripping apart of social order and the reestablishment of order via nonindigenous military forces.

The mental health worker may promote large-group identification by commenting not only on the shared emotional responses of victims but also on the courage, pride, and mutual support of the community. The media, especially television, are a remarkably effective means of encouraging group identity, as illustrated by the media-enhanced surge of patriotism in the United States during the 1991 Persian Gulf War. In essence, the mental health worker may use the media to present a highly condensed version of a large-group debriefing.

Clearly this approach must be balanced against the danger of becoming xenophobic. Ultimately, the traumatized community must reintegrate itself into the larger, nontraumatized society to restore healthy community identity.

Large-group debriefings.   The goals of large-group debriefings are

1. To promote a healing identification with the power and courage of the community at large by emphasizing that the entire community has suffered a trauma and that the entire community is in the process of recovery.
2. To normalize the emotions that individuals are experiencing and to provide a vocabulary for expressing their feelings to each other. This reduces the sense of isolation and helplessness that victims may feel.
3. To teach the audience simple self-help measures that can be used to relieve stress.
4. To educate the audience about when emotional responses may become destructive and professional help is indicated. Optimally, the sources of such help are also stated.

Debriefings encourage victims to respond to the disaster by talking about it, which has been reported to be the most common coping mechanism after a disaster (Wilkinson 1983). These debriefings may take a variety of forms. Terr (Chapter 5, this volume) described the "mini-marathon," which places a high emphasis on the expression of disaster experiences and emotions by each participant, usually within a 3-hour format. At times, organized groups will prefer a briefer, less self-revealing form of debriefing. The following is a description of a debriefing that is more didactic and less self-expressive than the mini-marathon and that can be delivered in approximately 1 hour.

The debriefing will have been initiated either by the group being addressed or by the debriefer. Optimally the debriefer will have some logical connection with the group, such as the parent of a school-age child who volunteers to debrief the school's parent-teacher association. This will foster the sense of "We're all in this together." If the debriefer is from outside the community, special sensitivity must be used to ensure that the audience does not feel as if they are being patronized or are on exhibition.

The debriefer opens the session by commenting that the group has shared a common disaster and that many of them may find themselves having powerful emotional responses. He or she may share personal experiences of the disaster or provide anecdotes given by others. The debriefer then will talk about the list of emotional reactions commonly experienced. It may be very helpful to mimeograph these lists and pass them out so that listeners may follow along. These lists are often then taken home, copied, and in turn distributed by listeners. The lists will vary according to the disaster, but may include those items listed in Table 3–1.

The debriefer talks about each of these symptoms, one by one, explaining each symptom and giving examples. Listeners will be encouraged to comment, question, or tell stories about their experiences with these feelings.

The debriefer then describes various forms of self-help. In particular, listeners are told that the single-best remedy for them is to be able to talk with each other about their feelings, experiences, and observations. "Talking about feelings allows us to relive the experience, but this time in a safer way, in the company of people whom we trust who are probably feeling exactly the same way," says the debriefer. "We can anticipate that we will all talk about the disaster, over and over and over again. Then, after time, without realizing it, we will notice that we are talking about it a bit less, and that healing has started to happen."

Other self-help measures to be stressed include spending extra time with family and loved ones. "Children are particularly vulnerable," says the debriefer. "Now, more than ever, just when you have so many other things on your mind, it's so important to take plenty of time with your kids, so they can talk about their scary feelings and feel the comfort of your love." The debriefer encourages the listeners to take extra time for recreation, to set limits on work and the pace of physically restoring one's home, and to allow oneself to lower standards for work productivity, obligations to others, or household responsibilities.

Table 3–1.   List of emotional reactions commonly experienced after a disaster

Anger	Fatigue	Nightmares
Apathy	Headaches	Numbness
Backaches	Helplessness	Over- or undereating
Boredom	Hopelessness	Poor concentration
Crying spells	Insomnia	Sadness
Difficulty with job performance	Intrusive thoughts	Shock
	Irritability	Substance abuse

"When all else fails, lower your standards," says the debriefer.

The debriefer then speaks of warning signs of stress reactions that require special attention. Behaviors such as increased use of alcohol, hurting one's children, significant weight loss, and severe insomnia are symptoms that may indicate that talking with a professional would be helpful. Symptoms in children such as nightmares, poor school performance, or prolonged regression to more childlike behavior indicate a need for professional help. Resources to obtain help should be specifically given. The "warning signs" as well as the mental health resources may also be noted on the handout. Finally, the debriefer opens the floor to comments and observations. Audience members vary widely in their ability to be open about their experiences, and preestablished group norms have great impact on the nature of dialogue between the debriefer and the audience.

If an entire large community has been traumatized, many debriefers will be required to reach all of the schools, churches, businesses, and organizations that may be interested in sessions. It may be very useful to provide several workshops to train debriefers and to maintain a "speaker's bureau" list of debriefers for interested groups.

Other recovery activities. Depending on the nature of the disaster, community, and the interests and talents of local mental health professionals, a variety of other recovery activities are possible. For example, the San Francisco Psychiatric Society established a telephone hot line to provide a listening ear for those traumatized by the earthquake (see Blaustein et al., Chapter 8, this volume). In some communities, mental health professionals may be asked to serve on local government disaster committees.

Certain groups requiring particular attention after a community disaster are trainees, such as medical students and residents who were affected by the disaster. Trainees often lack financial resources for quick recovery from a disaster. For example, some of our residents were renting homes that were completely destroyed during Hurricane Hugo and, lacking renter's insurance, lost all of their material possessions during the storm. Medical school and residency are difficult, stressful experiences under normal conditions. Obviously the stress of a disaster can be overwhelming. Many of our trainees also expressed concern that their training experience and certain critical rotations were significantly disrupted, and thought should be given to try to compensate for these disruptions. However, a disaster also provides a unique education opportunity for residents. Trainees have the chance to develop leadership skills as they are assigned important roles such as being in charge of a shelter or "pre-debriefing" a school.

Indigent people are an important group to reach who often remain outside traditional health care systems. Bolin and Lenow's (1988) research on psychological recovery after a tornado revealed that psychological recovery was positively correlated with socioeconomic status. Nontraditional sites of health care delivery must be considered to reach this subpopulation. For example, rural blacks living in marginal conditions without insurance were among the hardest hit by Hugo, and debriefings at churches proved to be the most effective means to reach this group. The problems of rural indigent people are compounded by the fact that small-town governments may be less aggressive and less successful at pursuing federal aid than big-city governments (L. Landon, personal communication, July 1990).

Elderly individuals compose another group potentially vulnerable to trauma. Disaster literature is inconsistent with regard to the effects of natural disasters on this population. Elderly people suffer disproportionate material losses (Bell 1976; E. Cohen and Poulshock 1975) and physical injuries during natural disasters and may also have poorer insurance coverage (Kilijanek and Drabek 1979). However, although some researchers suggest that elderly people are more likely to suffer emotional effects of a natural disaster (Erickson 1976; Moore and Friedsam 1959; Lifton and Olson 1976) than are younger people, other findings dispute this (Bell 1976; E. Cohen and Poulshock 1975; Hueta and Horton 1978; Kilijanek and Drabek 1979).

Although we have not yet analyzed our data on this point, our impression is that hurricane cleanup was particularly trying for elderly individuals but that this did not translate into a differential demand for traditional psychiatric services, perhaps reflecting continuation of patterns of lifelong nonuse of psychiatric services. We observed that although many of the elderly individuals were able to live independently as long as external circumstances were stable, negotiating with insurance companies and orchestrating major home repairs were beyond the capability of many. Some sustained injuries trying to clean and repair their homes. Many expressed discomfort at asking for help from grown children. Elderly individuals may wonder if their hometown will be restored to its former beauty within their lifetime. For some, a disaster was a reminder of painful existential realities, including the fragility and ultimate finality of life. It is obviously very important to include retirement communities and senior citizen centers in debriefings. During media interviews, one should remind listeners to take time to reach out to elderly friends, neighbors, and relatives.

Fortunately, in the case of large-scale disasters, federal and state agencies provide funding and human resources for mental health disaster response. For example, in response to Hurricane Hugo, the South Carolina Department of Mental Health established the Hugo Outreach Support Team, a group of trained social workers who fanned out into the community and provided debriefings and supportive counseling. This group was funded for 1 year after Hugo and made contact with more than 20,000 citizens by bringing care to the people at natural gathering places within the community. These disaster workers reported that the entrée to establishing a relationship with Hugo victims was first to address their needs for material supplies. In the process of addressing these concrete concerns, emotional issues were introduced gradually and nonthreateningly. The response to Hugo exactly paralleled experiences reported at other disasters: it is imperative to take clinical aid *to* the population at natural gathering places, rather than waiting for victims to come to traditional mental health care delivery sites (R. E. Cohen and Ahearn 1980).

Summary

In conclusion, the observance of several principles of disaster response may be useful in organizing an effective outreach to a traumatized community. Disasters unfold in a series of stages, each of which may require different types of interventions. Each disaster is unique, and the psychological reactions in the community may be powerfully affected by a variety of idiosyncratic issues and events. Large-group interventions may often be the treatment of choice, and the professional should, at a community level, attempt to enhance the individual's natural identification with the healing forces within the community. Finally, the therapist must take intervention to natural gathering places within the community, rather than assuming that victims will appear at traditional sites of mental health care delivery.

References

Austin L: In the wake of Hugo: the role of the psychiatrist. Psychiatric Annals 21(9):520–527, 1991

Bell W: Service Priorities for the Elderly in National Disasters. Omaha, NE, University of Nebraska, Gerontology Program, 1976

Berah E, Jones HJ, Valent P: The experience of a mental health team involved in the early phase of a disaster. Aust N Z J Psychiatry 18:354–358, 1984

Black JW: The libidinal cocoon: a nurturing retreat for the families of plane crash victims. Hosp Community Psychiatry 38:1322–1326, 1987

Bolin R, Lenow DJ: Older people in disaster: a comparison of black and white victims. Int J Aging Hum Dev 26:29–42, 1988

Cohen E, Poulshock S: The elderly in the aftermath of a disaster. Gerontologist 15:357–361, 1975

Cohen RE, Ahearn FL: Handbook for Mental Health Care of Disaster Victims. Baltimore, MD, Johns Hopkins University Press, 1980

Erickson K: Everything in Its Path. New York, Simon & Schuster, 1976

Ersland L, Weisaeth L, Sund A: The stress upon rescuers involved in an oil rig disaster, "Alexander L. Kielland," 1980. Acta Psychiatr Scand Suppl 355:38–49, 1989

Hueta F, Horton R: Coping behavior of elderly flood victims. Gerontologist 6:541–546, 1978

Kilijanek T, Drabek T: Assessing long term impacts of a natural disaster: a focus on the elderly. Economic Geography 47:438–451, 1979

Kinston W, Rosser K: Disaster: effects on mental and physical state. J Psychosom Res 18:437–456, 1974

Lifton R, Olson E: The human meaning of total disaster: the Buffalo Creek experience. Psychiatry 39:1–18, 1976

Mayfield M: Recovery from Hugo is slow, painful. USA Today, September 10, 1990, p 1

Moore H, Friedsam H: Reported emotional stress following a disaster. Social Forces 38:135–139, 1959

Quarantelli EL, Dynes RR: Images of Disaster: Myths and Consequences. Columbus, OH, Disaster Relief Center, Ohio State University, 1973

Rangell L: Discussion of the Buffalo Creek disaster: the course of psychic trauma. Am J Psychiatry 133:313–316, 1976

Raphael B: When Disaster Strikes: How Individuals and Communities Cope With Disaster. New York, Basic Books, 1986

Raphael B, Middleton W: Mental health responses in a decade of disasters: Australia, 1974–1983. Hosp Community Psychiatry 38:1331–1337, 1987

Tyhurst JS: Psychological and social aspects of civilian disaster. Can Med Assoc J 76:385–393, 1957

Weisaeth L: A study of behavioral responses to industrial disaster. Acta Psychiatr Scand Suppl 355:13–24, 1989

Wilkinson CB: Aftermath of a disaster: the collapse of the Hyatt Regency Hotel skywalk. Am J Psychiatry 140:1134–1139, 1983

Chapter 4

Training Mental Health Professionals to Work With Families in Diverse Cultural Contexts

Raquel E. Cohen, M.D., M.P.H.

*M*ental health intervention following disasters is becoming an important area of participation for mental health professionals (Ahearn and Cohen 1984). Its evolution has been influenced by national and international events that have highlighted the importance of psychological trauma in catastrophic life events. These events fall under several categories, including natural disasters, catastrophes caused by humans, and combinations of the two. The Three Mile Island radiation accident in March 1979 10 miles south of Harrisburg, Pennsylvania (Bromet 1980), the June 1972 destruction in two counties in Pennsylvania (Luzerne and Wyoming counties) by Hurricane Agnes, and the Buffalo Creek Valley, West Virginia, flood in February 1972 ("Disaster at Buffalo Creek" 1976; Gleser et al. 1981) are good examples of these categories. Although such disasters involve large numbers of individuals, national concern arises also for single individuals who are the victims of kidnapping or hostage situations.

If national expectations demand a well-trained cadre of mental health professionals, the form and requirements of such training must be determined. Such training must take into account the need to deal with diverse situations of multicultural societies that are affected by the disaster. This is especially true when the disaster occurs in an area where certain cultural groups congregate within small geographical boundaries, such as the tornado that devastated the town of Saragoza, Texas, in May 1987, an area inhabited primarily by Mexican American families.

In this chapter I address these cross-cultural issues. Certain components of high priority in the training of mental health professionals are emphasized.

The Caregiver

The training of mental health professionals must take into consideration the knowledge, attitudes, and skills arising from a diversity of cultural and educational backgrounds that they will bring with them. Cultural attitudes strongly influence the communication and response style of a disaster worker. These attitudes are deeply ingrained in the psychological systems of giving and asking for help. They also play a role in the psychology of victimization so that understanding and respecting the cultural values of the victims are part of the knowledge needed in disaster response.

These factors will have to be considered when designing a curriculum or practicum exercises. A simple questionnaire can be given to the workers, itemizing some key characteristics of their own cultural backgrounds. This will be helpful to the trainers developing the curriculum, who can then incorporate helpful guidelines addressing the interaction between the worker and the victim.

Role Definition

The role of the mental health professional within the postdisaster emergency relief agency staff is currently poorly defined (Cohen and Ahearn 1980). Mental health professionals are beginning to enter the well-organized governmental and Red Cross programs, which have operated for a substantial time in this field and which have already developed roles, responsibilities, and clear guidelines for responding to individuals who are victims rather than "patients."

The theoretical focus of the mental health professional must be shifted to a new system of guidelines that foster the development of knowledge, skills, and attitudes for working with individuals who are not sick, but traumatized. The evolution of such a role can already be found in some emergency trauma and hospital crisis units. The novel expectations of mental health professionals, both for themselves and others, can produce role discomfort and confusion.

Although professionals are sincere in their desire to assist victims, mental health workers are still not sure of their own and others' expectations regarding their activities. As they are trained, they should be prepared to adjust to the unfamiliar situations of emergency work in disasters and to develop methods of dealing with the reality of only minimal available data. Experience will help them to shift traditional attitudes in order to develop comfort and flexibility in collaborating with other disaster aid professionals. It becomes the task of the mental health team leader to define the mission and scope of the team's efforts and to communicate these to the team.

In working with colleagues from such agencies as the Red Cross, the Federal Management Agency, Civil Defense, and local law and rescue agencies, problems in certain areas may develop, such as disclosing confidential material, combining responsibility for mutual tasks, and respecting other value systems and communicating styles. Mental health workers may find themselves in conflict with long-standing traditions that guide the behavior of other disaster and emergency program workers. Often, the authority to make broad decisions rests with the lead government postdisaster agency. Some of these decisions may, at times, be made without consultation or consideration of the mental health implications for victims. Such events have produced problems for mental health professionals in their attempts to pursue collaboration and cooperation (Lystad 1988).

Role Configuration

Mental health workers are aware of status and professional behavior norms, which form a value system and "school of thought" within professional groups. In traditional clinical settings, professional boundaries are relatively clear, defining the structure and responsibilities of clinical services. A very different situation exists postdisaster, where there are enormous demands placed on mental health professionals in response to the needs of the community. The professional must set the limits and boundaries and prioritize the needs and resources as it becomes painfully clear that all needs encountered cannot be met. In this outreach situation, the mental health professional may be required to move from the role of "passive-receptive therapist" to "active-advocate mobilizer." As these role configurations develop, consideration must be given to the continuously shifting context in which the victims find themselves, reacting to abrupt relocation, differing shelter arrangements, and daily announcements of new directives from governmental authorities.

These constantly shifting scenarios change the mental health worker setting, demanding new, nontraditional mental health skills and attitudes. As both the public media and the governmental disaster assistance workers tackle major human issues and problems, they often turn to the "expert" for help. Such demands may include responding to newspaper reporters, participating on a television special, presenting a talk to school personnel, or acting as a consultant to the housing authority. These types of expectations from the community at large mold the role configuration of the disaster assistance personnel.

As workers become more experienced and comfortable with active outreach behavior, they may begin to anticipate needs and "invite themselves in" to become part of the community disaster response. This occurred in a community that had part of its city devastated by an ocean storm. The mental health worker phoned the medical reporter of the principal newspaper and suggested printing in the next edition a list of the expected psychological reactions to the disaster by age occurrence, so as to alert the readers and establish the fact that these were normal responses to a disaster. This list was printed in the next edition of the newspaper, and the responses of the public validated the helpfulness of the mental health approach.

The Victim

Many factors influence the degree of stress response experienced by a family system in a crisis, including the nature of the disaster (e.g., earthquake, hurricane, tornado, chemical spill), the type of property affected (urban or rural), and the community resources available for prevention and treatment of the secondary stressful effects of disorganized agency systems. Characteristics of the families affected, such as ethnicity, acculturation levels, socioeconomic status, value systems, and traditional methods of dealing with stressors, will also play a role in the recovery from the trauma. A particularly important value is the relationship of human beings to nature, which can be critical in understanding differences in the pattern of disaster response in diverse cultures.

For example, familiarity with the traditional kinship structure of Hispanic families (Kluckhohn and Strodtbeck 1961) shapes an understanding of how such individuals will respond to a disaster when facing issues such as search and rescue, providing aid to survivors, and sharing precious resources (e.g., food, water, and shelter). This understanding is necessary to develop organized mental health intervention programs. The Hispanic family is a kinship-oriented group and exhibits a reluctance to interact with the more formalized, nonkinship disaster operation approach with its shelters, organized work groups, and scheduled logistics.

Another social institution that must be considered together with cultural groups is organized religion. Religious groups are often involved organizationally in a wide scope of assistance activities, such as providing clothing, food, and shelter to victims, as well as providing traditional religious functions, such as burials and offering solace to the survivors.

The variability in form and severity of crisis reactions encountered by professionals working in a postdisaster situation presents a challenge to developing intervention approaches. The following example illustrates the multilevel activities developed to assist a family:

> Mr. Gonzalez, age 49, his wife, age 47, and their five children had recently immigrated to the United States from Honduras when a tornado damaged their home. Mrs. Gonzalez contacted the mental health team located in a church near the disaster site to ask for help to find out "if she was crazy." She met with the worker in the mental health team office and reported noticing that her feelings and behavior were changing. She had heard from neighbors that behavioral changes were to be expected after the trauma of the tornado. Despite this knowledge, she thought that her experiences went beyond the normal "posttraumatic reaction." She described feelings of depression, crying spells, and inability to make up her mind about household routines. She had no interest in anything and found it difficult to manage her children. Her normal social drinking had increased, and her friends had expressed concern about it.
>
> The family's home had been damaged, but they had already received financial assistance from government agencies, and workers were preparing to begin repairs. Although this component of the upheaval was proceeding in a satisfactory manner, the family was still experiencing serious troubles. Most of the wife's complaints and

expressions of difficulties centered on a husband who was suffering from multiple sclerosis, resulting in difficulty of movement and mood swings. Despite this disability, the husband wanted to control all aspects of the home's repair and the distribution of the funds received from government agencies. Mrs. Gonzalez felt her husband's attitude added to the complications associated with the repairs and thought he should be housed with relatives while the workers were in the house. Her marital situation, already shaky, had worsened, and she felt trapped. Although previously she had been able to function with strong, realistic defenses and with support from her friends and relatives, she now felt that everything was falling apart as her nearest family members had also suffered in the disaster and had been forced to move to other parts of the state.

The crisis intervention professional interviewed the husband, the couple, and the family to assess their psychological condition and hear their perceptions of the family's problems. She was able to perceive that the wife was using excessive control to deal with her feelings about the trauma, felt responsible for the problems that the family was having, and was unable to relinquish responsibility for the complex array of activities required. The ego capacity needed to handle the reality of her life and process the emotions resulting from the tornado and its effects was ineffective and had precipitated a crisis.

The professional also learned that the family's cultural tradition regarded the husband as the head and in control of the family, a role he did not want to relinquish. The professional, sensitive to this traditional value system, helped the wife to reassess and reevaluate her situation, showing her how the mix of traumatic events, traditional values, and her need for extended family ties were exacerbating the postdisaster crisis resolution process. By allowing Mrs. Gonzalez relief through verbal expression of her feelings, then guiding her into collaboration with her husband, rather than attempting to control his interactions with the repair workers, the professional helped her gain control of her emotions.

The wife was also helped to recognize her own internal feelings and how they remained a part of the unsolved and unfinished processing of the experiences of immigration and the subsequent disaster trauma. As Mrs. Gonzalez became aware of her increased efficiency, she began to feel more positive about her family. The worker supported her in her difficult reality situation and showed appreciation of her management of the bureaucratic requirements to get her home repaired despite her unfamiliarity with the "Anglo" procedures for obtaining the needed resources to assist her family after the disaster.

Such an example highlights the types of crisis intervention needed for victims after the basic, concrete postdisaster assistance is rendered to normalize living conditions. For many individuals, such assistance is not all that is required. The Gonzalez family had many problems before the tornado struck. The disaster unleashed latent problems in family relations, which were aggravated by the unresolved family crisis.

Basic Principles to Formulate Postdisaster Mental Health Intervention in a Multicultural Setting

How mental health problems are defined influences the interventions that are chosen and implemented. In the case of a postdisaster crisis reaction, one useful conceptualization is based on a bio-psycho-socio-cultural model of the individual's functions. The human crisis reaction that occurs in an individual after a disaster's sudden and intense impact is related to 1) age, gender, ethnicity, and economic status; 2) personality structure and usual coping defenses; 3) perception of stressor impact on his or her life; 4) the "fit" between the individual's needs and the availability of support systems; and 5) length of the period for resolution of the problems produced by the disaster. As the victim's biological, psychological, social, and cultural systems are affected, the victim strives to recover his or her usual level of functioning (Cohen and Ahearn 1980). The degree to which such processes succeed depends on many factors in the environment and within the individual. As the professional encounters the manifestations of human reactions to traumatic events, it is helpful to conceptualize the developmental phases of such manifestations (Cohen 1985).

The postdisaster sequences appear to be associated with the following psychological and emotional reactions.

Immediate Postdisaster State

The range of emotions expressed immediately after an individual realizes he or she is alive but traumatized by an event can include fear and anxiety, often masked by defenses such as denial and projection. Other emotions begin to appear as physical efforts become necessary to obtain safe shelter and knowledge regarding the location and condition of loved ones. Fear, anxiety, tension, and worry continue to manifest themselves, adding to the burden of the victims' wish for control as they struggle to survive and cooperate with the efforts of emergency assistance teams.

As time passes, behaviors change to show different ways of managing emotions, including many levels of depression produced by the victims' losses and changes of life-style. Frequent moves between temporary shelters may interfere with individuals' abilities to cope. Many cultural issues are raised by these living conditions, where individuals of different cultures are congregated and managed by an agency staff who have little knowledge of the victims' traditions or who may, themselves, be overwhelmed by their responsibilities and disruption of their own lives. An understanding of the variations and sequences of emotions and behaviors, based on cultural traditions and values, is at the heart of crisis intervention. Transcultural issues require modifications of aspects of crisis resolution processes that have been incorporated into clinical practice when dealing with "mainstream United States populations."

In disaster settings, the victims' self-esteem may be easily damaged as conflicts arise when victims' need to ask for help collides with workers' own beliefs about and skills in delivery of assistance. This conflict may be accentuated when victims perceive themselves as dependent on caregivers from a different culture or country. An empathic position is vital in responding to the victim's humiliation when forced to seek emergency supplies. These are but a few examples of situations that will influence the transculturally oriented configuration of the victim-helper (dependency-authority/power) relationship. Cultural traditions and values cut across all of these situations, affecting the amount of help that can be accepted or offered.

Postdisaster: Late State

The majority of the population will recover within 6–12 months after a disaster, returning to predisaster personality traits and social skills. Some victims may have difficulty reaching this normalization stage, presenting some of the pathological adjustments of chronic anxiety, mild to moderate depression, and difficulty with their jobs and family life. The degree of individuals' healthy adjustment will vary according to an array of variables interacting with characteristics of the disaster and the social aftermath.

This social aftermath, which is shaped by the victims' sociocultural context, interacts with 1) the victims' psychophysiologic reactions, 2) the emergency relief operations, 3) reconstruction efforts, and 4) the support and facilitation of crisis intervention programs. As time passes, the community regains its functional level. Organized religious activity is generally found in locations with large numbers of immigrant families, characterized by increased celebrations of reestablished rituals, including prayers for the dead and thanksgiving for the living.

Theoretical Basic Knowledge to Assist in Transcultural Crisis Intervention

Studies exploring the related problems of loss, mourning, separation, coping, and adaptation in families of different cultures in the United States are sparse (Sandoval and De la Roza 1986). A biopsychosocial intervention model in posttraumatic crisis stresses the individual's capabilities for adaptation, which develop in interaction with the family and community environment. Variations in coping styles are related to cultural "human programming" and psychophysiologic reactions to stressors. Although the area of research into reaction to catastrophic stressors in families of diverse cultural background is still evolving, and sufficient knowledge of the specific cultural repertoires of different families does not currently exist, awareness of the transcultural stance, sensitivity, and a need to obtain the victims' "worldview" of the situation are being addressed in the training of professionals working with such families in crisis (Szapocznik and Kurtines 1979). As we apply some of the knowledge obtained in different studies, the relationship of competence and socialization to attitude, self-esteem, and self-concept will affect postdisaster crisis resolution. These variables, supported by cultural mores and personality structure, will have an effect on the adaptive success of an individual's interaction within the environment of postdisaster reorganization.

Another area of importance having a bearing on many of the diverse cultural groups in the United States is the experience of "uprooting" (Coelho and Ahmed 1980). Uprooting, as a human experience, may be accompanied by depression and desolation. The same experience can, however, also offer a challenge, increasing coping and adaptation skills. As individuals are separated from their familiar social and cultural support systems, they are vulnerable to the consequences of change, while also challenged to develop different approaches to life patterns. The adaptation outcome may be an area of inquiry when working with a postdisaster multicultural population. It can be conceptualized by the interactions of vulnerability measures (migration and crisis), as reflected by the level of acculturation of the family and participation within the affected social environment after the disaster.

As a representative of a community effort, the mental health professional will be part of the influential organized postdisaster response of the community as it attempts to assist victims in an effective manner. By incorporating a transcultural intervention model, the professional will have the opportunity to anticipate and minimize the effect of the stressful situation produced by the disaster on an immigrant population. Components of the transcultural perspective are outlined in Table 4–1.

Summary

The training of mental health professionals for participation with their colleagues in postdisaster assistance work merits the attention of educational institutions. In the United States, all categories of mental health workers are learning to intervene and participate in postdisaster assistance work. Well-organized and operationally defined structures are already in place to help victims obtain shelter, food, loans, and medical help. The incorporation of mental health services, targeted to families of different cultures affected by a disaster, must be designed to match many of the special characteristics of the cultural norms of the group. Additionally, these services must be designed to interact with the organizational characteristics of the overall relief system, embodying rapidity of operations, flexibility of format, and collaboration and integration with the efforts of the other relief workers and service components.

Knowledge, skills, and attitudes for working with families of different cultures should be incorporated into the overall curriculum content of postdisaster training. The process of crisis resolution is influenced by internal and external factors, incorporating internalized value systems, role expectations, and traditional use of support systems and community resources. The multicultural living patterns of populations congregating in different parts of the United States (Los Angeles and Miami are good examples) necessitate adoption of a transcultural perspective for effective training of professionals working in the "front lines" of a disaster.

The techniques that should be modified and incorporated into postdisaster intervention are based on traditional skills. They differ substantially, however, in their application, according to 1) the intensity of the acute traumatic impact on the family and their "life space," 2) the complexity of interaction with professionals officially assigned by governmental relief operations who have the power to affect the families' lives dramatically, 3) the high ratio of families' needs to mental health resources, and 4) the novel, untried, unfamiliar, and conflicting roles of the crisis intervention professional in atypical disaster settings (e.g., shelters, damaged homes, motels, storefront offices).

Table 4–1. Components of the transcultural perspective

Cultural factors to be considered in crisis intervention

1. Migration and citizenship status—level of acculturation
2. Gender and parental roles
3. Religious belief systems
4. Child-rearing practices
5. Use of support systems (including extended family)

Clinical issues

1. Language dominance—assessment of use of language to ascertain reporting of symptoms, level of distress, and explanation of victim's "worldview"
2. Application of appropriate methodology to identify the cultural characteristics of the stressed family
3. Use of a transcultural frame of reference to interpret the crisis resolution behavior patterns of the family
4. Use of a transcultural methodology to organize the data obtained through different evaluation modalities (bio-psycho-socio-cultural) so as to identify the appropriate level of coping, crisis signs, dysfunction, or any DSM-III-R (American Psychiatric Association 1987) syndromes
5. Use of hypotheses, incorporating crisis theory and a transcultural perspective, to understand the influences bearing on coping and postdisaster adaptation as a final process of adaptation and resigation.

References

Ahearn FL, Cohen RE (eds): Disasters and mental health: an annotated bibliography (DHHS Publ No ADM 84-131). Washington, DC, U.S. Government Printing Office, 1984

American Psychiatric Association: Diagnostic and Statistical Manual of Mental Disorders, 3rd Edition, Revised. Washington, DC, American Psychiatric Association, 1987

Bromet E: Three Mile Island: Mental Health Findings. Pittsburgh, PA, Western Psychiatric Institute and Clinic and The University of Pittsburgh, 1980

Coelho GV, Ahmed PI (eds): Uprooting and Development. New York, Plenum, 1980

Cohen RE: Reacciones individuales ante desartres naturales. Boletin Oficina Sanitaria Panamericana (PAHO) 98:171–180, 1985

Cohen RE, Ahearn FL: Handbook for Mental Health Care of Disaster Victims. Baltimore, MD, Johns Hopkins University Press, 1980

Disaster at Buffalo Creek, Special Section. Am J Psychiatry 133:295–316, 1976

Gleser GC, Green BL, Winget C: Prolonged Psychosocial Effects of Disaster: A Study of Buffalo Creek. New York, Academic Press, 1981

Kluckhohn F, Strodtbeck F: Variations in Value Orientations. Evanston. IL, Row Peterson, 1961

Lystad M (ed): Mental Health Response to Mass Emergencies: Theory and Practice. New York, Brunner/Mazel, 1988

Sandoval MC, De la Roza MC: A cultural perspective for serving the Hispanic client, in Cross-Cultural Training for Mental Health Professionals. Edited by Lefley HP, Pedersen PB. Springfield, IL, Charles C Thomas, 1986, pp 151–181

Szapocznik J, Kurtines W: Acculturation, biculturalism and adjustment among Cuban Americans, in Psychological Dimensions on the Acculturation Process: Theory, Models, and Some New Findings. Edited by Padilla A. Boulder, CO, Westview Press, 1979, pp 139–159

Chapter 5

Large-Group Preventive Treatment Techniques for Use After Disaster

Lenore C. Terr, M.D.

*W*hen disaster strikes a community, a number of large-group preventive treatment techniques may be useful to address the psychological changes following the trauma. Shore et al. (1986), studying the Mount Saint Helens disaster in southwest Washington State in May 1980, reported that there are three mental disorders likely to affect a population after a catastrophic event: depression, generalized anxiety, and posttraumatic stress. Those individuals closest to the site of danger and destruction appear to stand the highest likelihood of developing a mental disorder. This appears to be true for children, too (Pynoos et al. 1987), although a new study of children's and adults' responses to a May 1988 Winnetka, Illinois, school shooting indicated that factors other than "dose of exposure" accounted for the development of posttraumatic stress disorder in this group (Schwarz and Kowalski 1991). A study of randomly selected, normal American schoolchildren 5–7 weeks after the Challenger space shuttle disaster of January 1986 demonstrated that the children's psychological reactions included fears; nightmares; visualizations; fantasies; supernatural experiences; creative attempts to handle anxiety through play, art, or writing; and changed attitudes about the self, the country, or the future (Terr et al. 1990). Fourteen months after the Challenger disaster, most of these attitudinal and philosophical changes continued to affect approximately the same percentage of children (Terr et al. 1990). The Challenger study demonstrated that normal populations of children and adolescents exhibit some internal mental changes after distant traumatic events, despite the fact that only a small number become clinically disordered.

Prevention must be aimed not only at those most likely to be traumatized, but also at those large groups who have been exposed to trauma. In this chapter, I discuss preventive and treatment techniques aimed at the very early emotional responses to disastrous external events. These interventions are aimed at preventing the development of psychological symptoms or frank disorders that may follow disasters.

Three large-scale group intervention models or techniques that can be used immediately after disaster are discussed: large-group psychotherapy techniques for groups of all ages, education interventions for children, and media (radio, television, and newspapers and magazines) techniques. The three kinds of immediate intervention are described, and some preliminary technical suggestions are offered. These modalities have been employed following recent disasters and seem to have significant potential for altering individual responses to terrible events.

Group Interventions

Mini-Marathon Sessions

At times of immediate and intense community need, group sessions for all age groups aimed at large, rather than small, groups of adults and children may be helpful. The idea of large-group debriefing sessions was initially developed for soldiers released from a war zone (Lifton 1973; Marshall 1947) and for hostages released by foreign terrorists (Rahe et al. 1990; Zimmerman 1983). The name *mini-marathon* sessions, originally coined by the psychologist Isaiah Zimmerman (1983), is used in this chapter for civilian groups that meet together after local calamities. I conducted three of these mini-marathons for civilians, for example, after the October 1989 San Francisco earthquake.

The objective of a mini-marathon session is to provide a structured 3-hour large-group session in which all participants are encouraged to speak. The session can be held anywhere from a living room to an auditorium. There is no intermission, but members are allowed to come and go. The participants may be from age 4 to the very elderly. Those younger than age 4 may attend, but they probably will not be called on to speak. If all have been exposed to the same event, then the group has enough in common to constitute a treatment group.

The mini-marathon session falls into three sections, each of equal importance: 1) sharing of stories from the event; 2) sharing of symptoms; and 3) sharing of positive stories of valor, future plans, and future solutions. If a second companion marathon session is planned, creative expression is elicited through drawing pictures with colorful markers or writing poems and then showing the pictures and reciting the poems. Good deeds from the past and expectations for the future conclude this second session.

Storytelling, an ancient art, is still an effective and interesting way to express feelings. "Each person," the leader says at the beginning of the mini-marathon, "knows a story of his or her own from the event that has just occurred. We are going to tell our own stories. Who wants to go first?" Everyone should be asked, and children in particular must be encouraged to speak. Thirty or more brief stories can be told. Even group members who do not choose to speak by the end of a session learn that, "We all went through this," "Most of us are bothered," and "We understand that some felt sad, some felt scared, and others felt wired, silly, and overexcited." The group leader, a mental health professional, accepts and validates all of these feelings. No expression of rage, excitement, titillation, or despair is invalidated by the leader. Terrible events stir up many types of responses, including a feeling of no emotional response in those inattentive or unmoved by the event or in those who were far from the center of the event. It is important, on the other hand, to reach those who feel numb but may be experiencing underlying, intense anxiety.

A goal of a mini-marathon group session is to prevent symptom development. Not all group members will have symptoms or are likely to develop symptoms. When providing preventive therapy, therefore, the leader anticipates and accepts the premise that some participants will go through the event without any symptoms.

The second part of the mini-marathon session is devoted to responding to symptom identification, symptom sharing, and the anticipation of future symptoms. The leader calls first for the most common symptoms, asking for a show of hands. "How many of you can see mental pictures of the earthquake as we speak?" "How many of you have already had a dream about it?" "How many of you feel afraid that another earthquake will strike?" The most common symptoms to affect a group exposed to disaster immediately are visualizations, trauma-specific fears, and dreams. Children may also express a need to sleep with someone else and to draw pictures of the disaster immediately after the event (Terr et al. 1990).

The leader discusses one symptom at a time with the group, beginning with visualization, because this finding is virtually ubiquitous. "Do any of you see yourselves standing or sitting in a certain position or a certain place?" the leader asks. The leader then allows the group to give instances of this. Systematic exposure and description of common symptoms and signs show group members the value of working therapeutically together. They are able to grasp the event in the context of peer responses. Children are asked to express themselves. The leader calls them by name or by description. Elderly persons are also, in particular, asked about their viewpoints. Elderly persons might tell of other earthquakes, other floods. Historical contexts—and the fact that elderly individuals are *here* to tell their stories today—are extremely helpful to the group. Geographical perspectives also help. The group realizes through the testimony of others that the disastrous incident or local tragedy has reached almost every one of them.

The leader then moves on to less ubiquitous, but very common, findings: dreams, fantasies, and fears. Each of these symptoms or responses should be shared by various members of the group. The leader asks if anyone has been inspired to do something creative related to the disaster. "Tell us about it," the leader says. "Show us." The leader then suggests how one might vary some of these creations. "There were other possible endings to what has happened here," the leader might say, if indeed there are other possibilities.

Toward the end of the second section of the mini-marathon session, the group leader mentions other psychological effects of the disaster that may appear in time: supernatural experiences, repetitive play, too much drawing or poetry, increasing fears, or changes in attitudes or philosophy. The leader explains that all of these are common responses, but when they occur they should be discussed with a trusted friend or family member. "We can help each other to stay healthy after disasters," the leader suggests, "by watching for signs that the disaster still is active in our minds. If a talk or two with a close friend or family member doesn't clear the fears, symptoms, or attitude changes, a member of my profession can be very helpful over a short period of time. Watch out for personality changes. These are signs that you will probably need some help." The mini-marathon leader thus instructs the group in how to identify those in need of professional help. Each member is also enabled to identify problematic behaviors in himself or herself.

The third part of the mini-marathon session, usually of shorter duration than the rest, consists of stories with optimistic themes, such as heroism, mastery of symptoms, or life after disaster. Any idea that can quench symptoms should be offered by the leader at this stage of the session. For instance, easy-to-use behavior modification techniques may be suggested for the group's most bothersome fears. Writing in journals, including dream journals, could be offered to those unaware of their feelings or too confused to verbalize them. Corrective denouements (Gardner 1971) may be useful to those overinvolved with pretend games and creative attempts. Aiding in community relief efforts may help reestablish for some group members a sense of being in control. Using "conscious dreaming techniques" (i.e., willing oneself in advance to "fix" the dream in a certain way) may offer relief from nightmares, especially if applied early in the postdisaster period (Garfield 1984).

At the end of the session, a heroic tale might be told by the leader—one, perhaps, that has been told before in the mini-marathon session but that can now be emphasized to achieve closure. A mini-marathon group meeting obviously includes considerable drama and ceremony. For large groups, drama and ceremony are major components of the tradition of dealing with disaster.

In this chapter I present a general and brief outline of mini-marathon group technique. My words should not be followed verbatim. I conducted three mini-marathon sessions with professional groups after the San Francisco earthquake. These groups—the Stanford Hospital House Staff, the staffs of two homes for runaway youth, and the consultants to several East Bay school systems—were led through the mini-marathon sessions so that they would be able to employ the very same technique in the places where they worked. When a psychiatrist introduces mini-marathons to other mental health professionals, he or she may reach many different subgroups in the community. One can conduct a mini-marathon session aimed at professionals while outlining to the group the three sections into which the session is divided and by explaining the key treatment aids that are being offered to the group: encouragement of abreaction; consensual validation; education; provision of peer, historical, and geographical contexts; and corrective denouement. The leader of a mini-marathon attempts to aid group members to resolve their shame and hidden responses. The leader also helps the group to anticipate and relieve symptoms and to identify those in need of psychotherapy.

A Note on Group Triage After a Disaster

In setting up smaller therapeutic groups after a disaster, individuals with similar backgrounds and experiences should be grouped together. If a number of deaths have occurred, those responding with both grief and shock should be grouped together regardless of age. Fornari (1991), for instance, ran several large-group meetings on Long Island in Spanish for the Avianca airplane crash survivors, their families, and some of the relatives of those killed. For more than a year after that disaster, Fornari's groups met in regularly scheduled sessions.

In groups for victims of sexual abuse, those abused in similar ways should be grouped together. Groups speaking foreign languages should be assigned to a therapist who speaks the same language. If members of a group are to go to court, leading questions and comments must be scrupulously avoided at group meetings. Exercises in hypnosis should not be taught or attempted (*Rock v. Arkansas* 1987). Such groups may be brought together for general discussions, but individual psychotherapy may also be necessary.

In cases of disaster where there are obvious legal problems, the attorneys representing members of the group should be consulted. However, in emergencies when the general public health is at risk, legal considerations are of lower priority than are health considerations. In large-scale community disasters, it is preferable to offer good prevention and treatment programs regardless of the possible later legal complications.

Educational Interventions

Schools are ubiquitous in America. If one wishes to reach children after community disasters or distant national events, one can reach them about 8 months a year at school. School-distributed media messages such as "Channel One TV" and *Scholastic News* carry public health messages into the world of children. The schools themselves, however, are a much more direct way to reach every child. Teachers and principals are able to speak with children face to face. They are able to answer directly individual children's questions and to serve as role models. School personnel may, at times, fill in for ineffective or absent parents.

In the past, schools made the mistake of not discussing community disasters with students. In attempting to avoid overexposure, a reasonable cause for concern, schools have habitually underexposed their pupils. For example, when the January 1989 Stockton, California, school shooting occurred, a Marin County principal less than 100 miles away ordered all the school's teachers *not* to mention the Stockton tragedy in class. The school was ordered into silence even though every newspaper, news program, and disc jockey in the area reported the incident.

What message is given when schoolteachers fail to discuss a nearby disaster? Among numerous possibilities are "Adults are afraid to talk." "Nobody knows what to do." "I'd better not bring this up at home—there's just something wrong about it." "Stockton must be something shameful."

Children need to learn as they grow up that the world is potentially dangerous and unpredictable. Life may end suddenly and prematurely. Bad luck exists but does not dominate life. These lessons—along with reading and math skills, history, geography, and literature—are the lessons that schools must teach. The lessons children learn regarding psychological responses to distant tragedies stimulate their emotional growth so they are able to exist and travel in the world. If children are forced to learn these lessons all alone in urban ghettos, they may develop beyond strength toward a calloused position. If, on the other hand, children learn these lessons only at home from their parents, they may become overly sensitive to small nuances from personal and distant events.

Schools, at times, may blunder into overexposures or harmful exposures of their pupils. One North Carolina teacher, for instance, in discussing a babysitter who attacked and shot children in a Winnetka, Illinois, elementary school classroom, pointed out that her own third-grade students were too noisy and unruly—she could not have given them "the proper signals" if a crazed, gun-toting person had come into her classroom. This teacher's students, of course, struggled to behave properly after hearing their teacher's well-intentioned, but destructive, comment. They obeyed while paying the price of their own increased anxiety.

The superintendent of schools at Stockton, California, allowed the popular rock star Michael Jackson to visit Cleveland Elementary School a few weeks after that school suffered an attack by a man shooting a semiautomatic weapon. Michael Jackson's visit was to be a form of consolation prize. The school population was 75% Southeast

Asian, most of whom were recent immigrants. The rock star arrived in the school yard by helicopter, accompanied by police cars with flashing blue lights and sirens and uniformed police officers. The shooting itself had been accompanied by the same flashing blue lights, uniforms, and helicopter noise. Many students panicked. "Another bad man," they screamed. "More ambulances." The teachers assured them it was "Michael Jackson, Michael Jackson." "Who is Michael Jackson?" the children inquired, still confused. They were not familiar with rock music or rock stars and could not appreciate Michael Jackson's and the school superintendent's ill-directed gifts to them. Ironically, the school superintendent did not allow mental health workers to conduct research in her schools the year after the shootings, saying that it would take too much time away from education.

Disaster Programs for Schools

The first step in planning the response of schools after disasters or international events is to establish a preexisting, warm, open consulting relationship between mental health professionals and the schools. Psychiatrists and other mental health professionals should regularly interact with schools in planning for disasters, establishing research projects, and delivering services. Each traumatic situation is different. Each situation requires mental health services from the very beginning, not at the end.

Schools may use ceremony to help large groups of children to process frightening events. If a child from the school is killed over the summer holiday in an automobile accident or dies of acquired immuno-deficiency syndrome, most children already know about it when school starts. Rumors travel quickly among children. Uninformed children find out about tragedy soon enough, once school starts. Such a tragedy may be appropriately responded to with a moment of schoolwide silence for the child. Teachers of classes in the dead student's grade should talk with their pupils about the child.

The end of a war is cause for schoolwide celebration. Happy outcomes call for anything from a singing assembly to a hot dog roast. While the children are celebrating, balance may be brought to the occasion. The principal might pray for our dead soldiers, or a child's poem might be dedicated to a lost hostage. Just as ceremony marks death and schoolwide tragedies, so too ceremony marks the end of stress and the beginning of optimism. One or two ceremonies a year might help schools bring the real world into children's lives.

The classroom, however, is where children "live" much of the time, and most good can be done directly in class. Children should be asked by their teachers to discuss an event that has upset the people in the town. Other children may respond and share their feelings together. The teacher can summarize the situation, clarify facts, and offer solace. Everything said must be truthful. No false reassurances or scapegoating should be offered.

Once a short discussion has taken place in the class, children may be asked to draw their own pictures, paint a giant cooperative work of art, write poems or letters to pen pals, compose rhyming couplets for "rap" music, participate in creating a television tape, or prepare a small skit. Any kind of creative effort, especially when informal and not requiring rehearsal or polished performances, will help youngsters gain control of the intense emotions and sense of helplessness that follow community disaster. The children in a classroom can show their creative work to other youngsters, sharing feelings and offering experiences to their peers.

The teacher may also use such exercises to identify children in need of professional help. For example, if a child draws a picture of a dying grandmother in the course of a group project around Saddam Hussein, that child may be showing the teacher he is overwhelmed by tragedies far nearer to home. The teacher should then consult the mental health services of the school about that particular child. In general, however, classroom exercises such as those described are often sufficient to reassure the child. Adding corrective denouements (Gardner 1971) is a helpful ending to a classroom discussion. "How can we settle the problems that follow the war in Iraq?" the teacher might ask toward the end of a classroom session. "Is there anything we can learn from Danny's tragic accident?"

When an unsettling film, such as *Nightmare on Elm Street* or *Halloween* is popular among youngsters, interested teachers might consider seeing the film and later discussing it with students. Such films have terrified millions of children. Similarly, when certain unsafe fads infect groups of adolescents, group techniques at school might be considered. Teen suicide, however, remains an uncertain area for school intervention because further suicides may be stimulated if the mental illness behind the adolescent suicide is not carefully pointed out (Shaffer et al. 1990).

Adolescents prefer to use sophisticated creative equipment—air brushes and acrylic paints instead of poster paints, for example, or the electronic synthesizer rather than a piano—when they create together as a group. The need to do something creative remains high in adolescence, especially after community disasters. Rap songs, handmade television "commercials," poetry, letters, and journals are popular with teens. These techniques can be used to facilitate communications, expression, and learning. What, after all, is more important for children and youth than to learn how to cope creatively with life's events?

For further description and discussion of school interventions, the reader is referred to Eth (Chapter 6, this volume).

The Media

Radio

Immediately after the San Fernando Valley, California, earthquake of the early 1970s, a social agency went "on the air." The agency put together a call-in radio talk show that provided a community sounding board for those phoning in and those listening to their radios. The agency social workers not only let people express themselves, but they also made preventive and treatment suggestions (Blaufarb and Levine 1972). The radio audience was able to have their feelings consensually validated by their peers in the community. They learned that others were affected but were coping.

Joining a similarly affected peer group has been proven to help people other than disaster victims; examples include cancer psychotherapy groups (Spiegel et al. 1989) and Alcoholics Anonymous. The knowledge that it is not abnormal to be affected by a disaster appears to help victims of terrible events. Knowing that others also felt helpless relieves shame and restores dignity. Adolescent suicide is the sole exception to this truism about peer group support. Teen suicide has been shown to be precipitated by television news announcements of adolescent suicides (Phillips and Carstensen 1986) and perhaps by fictional television shows about teen suicide (Gould and Shaffer 1986). Suicide epidemics, however, represent negative fallout from a form of intervention that, in many important instances, is potentially positive.

Radio talk shows offer the chance for particularly effective immediate communication within communities besieged by disaster.

These talk shows should generally be broadcast during hours when everyone, children and elderly people alike, is able to participate. The programs may be aired immediately in the wake of a disaster. Mental health professionals from the community are the most appropriate persons to operate the phone lines. Surgeons, police officers, and others with special knowledge and skills may participate, if their particular expertise is needed. Experts on childhood responses and on the problems of aging may be available to answer questions from these specific groups. Information about planned individual and group psychotherapeutic interventions should be announced during these radio talk shows. It is important for agencies contributing to talk shows to follow through with their promised interventions.

Specialized radio talk programs may be oriented to certain special groups in the community. Postdisaster radio talk shows may be developed for teenagers in association with locally popular disc jockeys. In the event of a disaster in Zuni or Navaho country, "talk" opportunities might be established for Native American children on reservation music programs that ordinarily play traditional chants and rock music. The mental health professional determines the target groups that are most likely to be affected by a certain event and then gears "talk radio" toward these groups. The 1989 Cleveland Elementary School shooting in Stockton, California, which affected mainly Southeast Asian children, may illustrate this point. On Stockton radio programs in the Hmong, Cambodian, and Vietnamese languages, the Southeast Asians affected by the disaster would potentially have been immediately reachable. The ordinary American disc jockey or radio talk show would have missed the most severely affected group after this particular school disaster.

Radio talk shows, once established as community outreach programs during and after large-scale disastrous events, should continue daily for several days. They should allow for ongoing interaction between callers and mental health professionals. These talk shows should also advertise the mental health treatment programs that will be provided for individuals and small groups. It may be necessary for representatives of the psychiatric and psychological associations to pay site visits to the treatment programs that will be suggested by radio talk show hosts. One must ensure that they are 1) in existence, 2) ethical, 3) following established treatment techniques, and 4) consistent with the standards operative in the community.

Print Media

Although books and magazine articles are excellent ways to educate the public about disaster on a thorough or scientific basis, newspapers are an excellent way to reach the public almost immediately. Print has one distinct advantage over radio: it lasts. Newspapers can be consulted several times a day and by several members of one family. Newspapers may be saved and even clipped to a bulletin board or refrigerator. Mental health professionals may submit articles to newspapers for publication, usually in the form of editorials or letters to the editor. More often, professionals can reach the public quickly through interviews with news or science reporters from the regular newspaper staff. Mental health professionals should acquaint themselves with the news, science, or psychology writers in their community. After disaster strikes, contacts that were made under conditions of calm can immediately be turned to the purposes of public mental health prevention and treatment. If trusting relationships with the press are formed in advance, it is more likely that accurate and helpful information will be released by the local newspapers during times of disaster.

It would be advisable for local mental health societies to keep funds available to take out newspaper ads at the time of community mental health emergencies. Effective therapeutic programs responding to a disaster could be described and explained to the public in such advertisements.

Letters to the editor of widely circulated newspapers allow professionals quick, direct access to the public during disastrous or frightening times. The following is an example of one such letter (Terr 1991) published in the *New York Times* during the Persian Gulf War:

First, How Do Children Feel About the War?

To the Editor:

"What Should Be Taught About War in the Gulf?" (Education page Jan. 23) takes the premise that our schools should be teaching children better factual lessons about the Middle East. But intense feelings by students obscure their ability to understand or use the facts.

I am a psychiatrist, working with children and adolescents, who studies trauma. In a study of 152 randomly selected children in the United States after the Challenger space shuttle exploded five years ago, I found that 19 youngsters who had not had the chance to respond to a 45-minute, structured interview given five to seven weeks after the disaster were not doing as well in 1987 as the 133 children who had completed this first interview. This means that by simply talking to a friendly adult about a distant disaster, children are not as likely to suffer from grief and terror.

There have been outbreaks of mass hysteria several times in world history. Saddam Hussein might wish for the world of children to engage in mass hysteria right now. Questions about bombs, threats of chemical warfare and terrorism, when left silently unexpressed and therefore unanswered, hold the potential for major psychological distress in the world of children. If children are not given the opportunity to speak of such concerns as nuclear attack, terrorism, and germs openly at school with teachers, they will not be open to the facts all of us hold so important.

I would suggest that we first let American schoolchildren express themselves about the Persian Gulf War. Creativity, as in art work, poems, television rap commercials and dramatizations, can be extremely helpful, especially when these productions are not rehearsed and re-rehearsed for ultimate delivery in an auditorium. Later the facts will be absorbed with more open minds and more friendly hearts. Kids need historical and geographical contexts in which to place their emotions.

A 5-year-old told me today she was worried about the gulf bombings. "What worries you about it?" I asked. "That Jordan will be bombed," she said. I could have said, "Jordan's not in this war" and offered the "fact" that Jordan's not in any danger. I chose instead, "What is it about Jordan that frightens you?" She answered, "My brother." Her younger brother's name was George. Her worry—the connection—was the sound of her brother's name.

We will not be able to offer kids the right facts until we know their feelings.

Lenore Terr, M.D.
San Francisco, February 1, 1991
[Terr is the author of
*Too Scared to Cry:Psychic
Trauma in Childhood* (1990).]

Television

Television "interventions" at times of disaster are quite different than those of radio or the newspapers. Typically, the television news show about a community disaster allows the mental health professional only one or two "sound bites" in which to offer helpful statements. He or she must use this opportunity to express the single most important point. Preparing this statement in advance is advisable. It may be useful to express this point with colorful metaphor.

Television emphasizes visual appearance rather than deeper realities. Friendly, warm interactions with the interviewer help the mental health professional look good in the public's "eye." When the viewer considers accepting or rejecting the help being offered on television, this warm, friendly approach may make the critical difference.

Local and national television talk shows and educational shows are prearranged through producers. Producers determine the program format, guests, and focus of the show. The producer will edit the material. It is important to discuss matters of production with the producer early in the course of the program planning. It is also important to decide actively whether or not to join the show that is being proposed. Consideration of mental health's primary goals—public prevention, education, and intervention—will help to decide if the proposed show may help achieve those goals. The television industry obviously has many other goals, although the above three are among them. When there is agreement between disciplines about goals, mental health professionals will benefit their communities and the nation by appearing on television. Clearly television reaches an enormously wide audience.

It is important that the mental health professional learns to "master the media." Statements, whether spontaneous or prepared, must be short and must convey a single point in the most colorful language possible. Relatively indirect answers to an interviewer's questions are acceptable on television if they lead to an important point. Both men and women may have to apply their own face makeup to appear before the strong lights and probing lenses of the television cameras. Television destroys the tired or the bedraggled. It is important to look wherever the camera operator suggests and to maintain a steady gaze even if no person inhabits that space. It helps to imagine a friendly listener behind the lens or behind the wall if one's eyes are fixed on it. Smiles, whenever appropriate, convey the pleasant appearances so necessary to television communication. For further discussion of these principles, the reader is referred to Ruben (Chapter 7, this volume).

On television, the mental health professional must stay unruffled in the presence of other professionals with opposite points of view. The "process" of television is often its major message. Experts can disagree pleasantly without bickering. The most important point that the public must learn is that competent professionals are available to help them through an emergency. The process of television may be "staged," but the message of competence, capability, and willingness to accept responsibility must always be conveyed. The public is extremely interested in health maintenance and in stress management. Although the public may avoid facing information about severe mental disorders, people are extremely interested in knowing how they might stay mentally healthy (Yankelowich 1991). This public interest in health should be the focus at times of disaster.

Psychiatrists can be useful to television and film scriptwriters who are planning films and features about mental responses to catastrophes. When psychiatric consultants help plan fictional depictions of these responses, the results are more true to life and the audience is able to anticipate how they would respond after a disaster. Practice is an effective aid to coping. Those who have experienced Army basic training confirm that training provides immunization to psychic trauma. Pretending offers coping options for future events. The public learns without really knowing that it is being taught. For instance, when Dustin Hoffman portrayed an autistic "savant" in the film *Rainman,* Peter Tanguay, a well-known psychiatric expert on autism, helped both the scriptwriter and the actor prepare. The result was a film that educated and enabled the public to empathize with a serious mental disorder (Vanderweit 1991).

Children represent an audience that has not yet been effectively reached by radio or television at times of disaster. A commercial television station for children, Channel One, operates in many American high schools and offers news and feature stories oriented to children's emotional and intellectual needs. Some interesting "spot" announcements have helped children with kidnapping threats and wartime worries. However, very few techniques have been developed for younger children to provide mass prevention, education, and treatment at times of public emergency.

During the Persian Gulf War, two national news networks attempted to reach younger children on Saturday morning, January 26, 1991. Regularly scheduled cartoon hours were canceled. Unfortunately, neither program effectively handled the questions children asked on the toll-free lines. News correspondents in the field spoke directly to their own anchor, rather than to the children who called. The reporters spoke in three-syllable terms about such things as "political versus military solutions," "the eye of the beholder," and "national images." They spoke very slowly, perhaps on the assumption that slowly delivering multisyllable, abstract language to children under age 12 would make the complex wording and thought understandable. Children shown in the audience of one program fretted, fussed, yawned, and looked distracted. One child asked about something he found frightening, the danger of SCUD missiles. The responding journalists offered even more frightening information, saying that the SCUDs were not as dangerous as the nuclear, chemical, and germ warfare that could be unleashed at any time. Reporters volunteered extra details that children did not want or need to know. For instance, children were told that chemical warfare caused blisters all over the body or an "overload of the nervous system" that would eventually cause a person to become "paralyzed and then die." In one instance, a young girl's motives for asking a question about a future military draft were called into question by the presiding news anchor. "Somebody put you up to this," the anchor said. The child responded that she had two teenage brothers. "Ah ha, I *knew* somebody put you up to this," the anchor replied.

The two national news programs for children of January 26, 1991, were viewed by millions of American youngsters. The programs clearly had been constructed without effective child psychiatric or psychological consultation. Child psychiatrists did not appear on television and apparently had not been consulted at the time of production. If television is to be effective during times of disaster, psychiatrists must help with program development as consultants. During the delays preceding the broadcasting of individual audience questions, mental health professionals would "translate" the child's words for the anchor and help develop responses to the caller's question. The public needs to be allowed to express the feelings and worries behind their questions. What about the SCUDs bothered American youngsters? Why were they so concerned about the military draft? How did children think that chemical warfare would affect them? Did they know any children who had temporarily been orphaned because two parents were serving in the Gulf War? Was the audience concerned about ecological disaster when oil spilled out into the Gulf? Did children have a guess about how many wars we have fought since their parents were born?

The goal of mass media interventions at times of war should be to allay fears and to offer understanding of the context of the war. Child audiences need to express their feelings first and to learn the facts later. Children may be allowed to show their artwork and poems on television, to sing their songs, and to share their feelings with other children in other places. Their fears will be reduced by learning the contexts— geographical, historical, and literary—in which wars occur. By establishing an understanding of context, children can integrate their fears into a far broader perspective than they would otherwise know.

Short television spots for children appeared to be more relevant to their concerns than was the major network television news during the Persian Gulf War. Brief commercial-like spots on the public broadcasting channels featuring Mr. Roger's promise, "Somebody will be there to take care of you [my paraphrase]" gave very young preschoolers reasonable reassurances. One 10-year-old girl commented that "Kids' Town News," a 2-minute spot that is shown during the late afternoon in her city, had helped her. "One neat thing about the war," she said, "they showed weird facts on 'Kids' News.' They showed children who went there [to the Middle East] and got a mask, a coin, and a thing that protects your hands [from poison gas]. The kids [they showed on television] were somewhere around Iraq, but not *in* there. The Iraqis dumped the oil and killed the animals—I saw it on TV. I read it in *Scholastic News*; and 'Kids' Town News' has two minutes of unboring facts, like those kids who went someplace in the Middle East and then talked about it." This 10-year-old girl benefited from short television spot programming because she was shown pictures of her peers and of things that automatically interest children. She learned more in that context than she could learn from the ordinary television news broadcast.

Summary

Three broad areas for large-group interventions and preventions in disaster-struck communities have been described, discussed, and reviewed in this chapter. Mini-marathon sessions, educational interventions for children, and media interventions (radio talk shows, newspaper writing, television programs, and films) reach large numbers of individuals experiencing severe stress. Further research will explore the usefulness of these interventions. As mental health professionals participate in mass group interventions, expanded techniques will be developed to respond to community and national disasters.

References

Blaufarb H, Levine J: Crisis intervention in an earthquake. Social Work 17(7):16–19, 1972

Fornari V: Team treatment approach for disaster survivors: Avianca plane crash. Presented at the annual meeting of the American Academy of Child and Adolescent Psychiatry, October 1991

Gardner R: Therapeutic Communication With Children: The Mutual Storytelling Technique. New York, Science House, 1971

Garfield P: Your Child's Dreams. New York, Ballantine, 1984

Gould M, Shaffer D: The impact of suicide in television movies. N Engl J Med 315:690–693, 1986

Lifton R: Home From the War. New York, Basic Books, 1973

Marshall SLA: Men Under Fire. New York, William Morrow, 1947

Phillips D, Carstensen L: Clustering of teenage suicides after television news stories about suicide. N Engl J Med 315(11):685–689, 1986

Pynoos R, Frederick C, Nader K, et al: Life threat and post-traumatic stress in school-age children. Arch Gen Psychiatry 44:1057–1063, 1987

Rahe R, Karson S, Howard NS, et al: Psychological and psychosocial assessments on American hostages freed from captivity in Iran. Psychosom Med 52:1–16, 1990

Rock v Arkansas, 483 US 44:107 S Ct 2704, 97 L Ed 2d 37, 55 US LW 4925, 1987

Schwarz ED, Kowalski JM: Posttraumatic stress disorder after a school shooting: effects of symptom threshold selection and diagnosis by DSM-III, DSM-III-R, or proposed DSM-IV. Am J Psychiatry 148:592–597, 1991

Shaffer D, Vieland V, Garland A, et al: Adolescent suicide attempters: response to suicide-prevention programs. JAMA 264:3151–3155, 1990

Shore JH, Tatum EL, Vollmer WM: Psychiatric reactions to disaster: the Mount St. Helens experience. Am J Psychiatry 143:590–595, 1986

Spiegel D, Bloom JR, Kraemer HC, et al: Effect of psychosocial treatment on survival of patients with metastatic breast cancer. Lancet 2:888–891, 1989

Terr L: Too Scared to Cry: Psychic Trauma in Childhood. New York, Harper & Row, 1990

Terr L: Letter to the editor. New York Times, February 22, 1991

Terr L, Bloch D, Michel B, et al: Children's responses to the Challenger disaster (New Research Abstracts). Paper presented at the annual meeting of the American Psychiatric Association, New York, May 13–17, 1990

Vanderweit J: Child psychiatrist consults for the movies. American Academy of Child and Adolescent Psychiatry Newsletter, Spring 1991, p 35

Yankelowich D: Public attitudes about psychiatric disorder and mental health. Paper presented as the Doctor John Adams Memorial Lecture, American College of Psychiatrists, Ft. Lauderdale, FL, February 9, 1991

Zimmerman I: Adaptation to terrorism and political violence. Paper presented at the annual meeting of the Los Angeles Group Psychotherapy Society, Los Angeles, CA, June 1983

Chapter 6

Clinical Response to Traumatized Children

Spencer Eth, M.D.

*A*longside our society's romantic vision of childhood as a happy time of carefree pleasures is the stark reality that many children face a life filled with stress and trauma. Fortunately, children seem to enjoy a remarkable capacity to overcome adversity. However, even the most resilient child may become symptomatic in the aftermath of a particularly disturbing event. In this chapter I first explore the psychopathological consequences for children of community disaster and then describe one form of therapeutic intervention of particular value in responding to major traumas. This technique, which involves a school-based group consultation, has been employed successfully after a variety of traumatic events and may serve as a model of the type of efficient and economical mental health service that is necessary after a disaster has struck.

Psychopathological Responses to Stress

Although many psychiatric conditions in childhood may be related to or exacerbated by stress, two specific disorders defined in DSM-III-R (American Psychiatric Association 1987) are actually caused by disturbing life events such as a community-wide disaster (Turkel and Eth 1990). Adjustment disorder and posttraumatic stress disorder (PTSD) refer respectively to the milder and more severe syndromes etiologically linked to stress and trauma. DSM-III-R defines adjustment disorder as a pathologic reaction to an identifiable psychosocial stressor that occurs within 3 months and lasts less than 6 months. The maladaptive nature of the reaction is indicated by an impairment in school or social function and by symptoms that are in excess of a normal reaction to that stressor. DSM-III-R lists nine subtypes of adjustment disorder according to whether the predominant symptom affects emotions, conduct, schoolwork, and/or physical or social function. There is no typical clinical picture of adjustment disorder in childhood, and the reaction to stress depends on many variables. Further, it is often difficult to define clearly the thresholds of the maladaptive and symptomatic responses that constitute adjustment disorder in children and to predict the likely course of the condition. However, in general, the prognosis for this condition is favorable as it comprises those children with fewer and milder symptoms than the group with PTSD.

PTSD refers to the cluster of symptoms that characteristically appears after an extremely disturbing life event, which is by definition outside of the range of usual human experience and would be markedly distressing to almost anyone (American Psychiatric Association 1987). Despite differences in the nature of the precipitating event, a wide range of psychosocial stressors, including natural disasters, accidental injuries, and acts of violence, can produce similar psychological consequences. Although the early scientific literature ascribed PTSD to frank brain injury, it is now accepted that the etiology is psychogenic, and the condition is classified as one of the anxiety disorders (Eth et al. 1989). The hallmarks of PTSD are the core symptoms of reexperiencing the trauma, psychic numbing, and increased psychophysiologic arousal. Recurrent, intrusive, and painful memories and dreams are common manifestations of reexperiencing phenomena. Of equivalent diagnostic significance for younger children is traumatic play, in which elements of the event are reenacted in a repetitive, stereotyped, and joyless fashion. In rare instances, dissociative states, flashbacks, or hallucinatory reliving of the trauma may be seen. Children are prone to distress when exposed to events that symbolize or resemble an aspect of the trauma or on the anniversary of its occurrence.

Psychic numbing refers to a group of related symptoms that range from an isolated inability to remember an important feature of the trauma to a pervasive erosion of interest in life, which in very young children may present as a regressive loss of acquired skills, such as expressive language. Psychic numbing may also be seen as constricted affect, interpersonal detachment, and pessimism about the future. Another psychological means to minimize the distress of remembering is by persistent avoidance of reminders of the trauma. Suppression of thoughts and feelings and attempts to avoid activities or situations reminiscent of the traumatic event are common, although usually unsuccessful, efforts to control the distress intrinsic to the disorder. The final cluster of symptoms that permits the diagnosis of PTSD are the indicators of pathologic psychophysiologic arousal. Irritability, hypervigilance, exaggerated startle reactions, and poor concentration are readily observable and contribute to the appearance of nervousness. Not surprisingly, anxious trauma victims have difficulty falling asleep and staying asleep.

It should be recognized that there are important differences in symptomatology as a function of the nature of the specific traumatic event and of the characteristics of the particular child (Terr 1991). Although there is no universally agreed on or obviously fundamental taxonomy of disasters, several salient variables have been identified (Kinston and Rosser 1974). Traumatic events vary with regard to their 1) origin, 2) speed of onset, 3) social preparedness, 4) duration, 5) scope of impact, 6) proportion of persons affected, 7) degree of life threat and suffering, and 8) potential for reoccurrence. It would seem that sudden, unexpected, human-induced events that cause widespread death and destruction have greater "traumatogenic" potential. The susceptibility of an individual child to a psychosocial stressor is the product of several factors. The child's genetic, constitutional, and temperamental endowments, as well as any medical and psychiatric comorbidities, are relevant in assessing vulnerability. Other risk factors include the presence of previous exposure to traumatic events and the state of mind at the time of the incident. The adequacy of the child's coping skills and the ability of the parents and community to offer support are important posttrauma considerations.

Age-Specific Differences

There are notable differences in phenomenology of the traumatic syndrome according to the developmental phase and age of the child (Eth 1990). The earliest recognizable traumatic syndrome may be seen in the 30- to 36-month-old child; before that age the child has difficulty encoding and retrieving verbal memories of traumatic experiences, and the resulting symptoms are nonspecific (Terr 1988). More than any other age group, preschool children can initially appear as withdrawn, subdued, or even mute. This stance should not be mistaken for amnesia since the child may later choose to reveal the details of the traumatic incident to a loved one. Young children are prone to regression in the wake of a trauma. Anxious attachment behavior, intensified separation and stranger anxiety, temper tantrums, and a return to the use of transitional objects are emblematic of the early response of the traumatized preschooler. Stage 4 sleep disturbances, such as somnambulism, sleep talking, night terrors, and restlessness, are common.

Whereas preschool children engage in solo play around traumatic themes, school-age children may also involve their friends in redramatizations and trauma-related games. The school-age child exhibits a wider range of cognitive, behavioral, and emotional responses to traumatic events (Eth and Pynoos 1985). Schoolchildren often display features of cognitive constriction, which may present as a functional impairment of intellectual performance in class. The child's declining ability to concentrate derives from a combination of factors, including distraction by the intrusion of traumatic memories, inhibition of spontaneous thought consistent with an evolving cognitive style of forgetting, and interference from anxious and depressed affects. Children 6–12 years old may also be preoccupied with various aspects of the traumatic situation. Some children fantasize about how they might have acted differently before, during, or after the trauma. In these fantasies children may imagine having extraordinary power that enables them to prevent damage or rescue survivors. Where human-induced violence has been causative, the child might elaborate gruesome revenge fantasies, which may serve to relieve the child's guilt over not having been able to do more at the time.

Some children spend an inordinate amount of time reporting the traumatic incident to anyone who will listen. By so doing, the child is employing the latency defense of isolation of affect by obsessively fixating on the details of the trauma to the exclusion of feelings. The reverse is also possible, where the child remains in a perpetual state of anxious arousal, as if to prepare for imminent danger. This hypervigilance may permit the child to substitute memories of the past trauma with self-initiated fantasies of future threat.

In school, traumatized children can display a diversity of behavioral symptoms. Normally placid students may become irritable, rude, and provocative; exuberant children may become inhibited and withdrawn. As a result, peer relationships will suffer, especially if a child becomes aggressive, moody, or unpredictable. Children may be aware of these changes and then react with a loss of self-esteem and self-confidence.

Children can experience intense perceptual sensations during a traumatic event. Depending on the nature of the event, any or all sensory modalities may be activated. In addition, the child may notice unpleasant feelings associated with autonomic arousal. Traumatized schoolchildren seem particularly prone to the development of psychosomatic complaints, such as headaches and stomach pains. After a disaster, visits to the school nurse and pediatrician may be expected to multiply, even among otherwise healthy children. Various explanations for this phenomenon have been offered, including resomatization of affect and identification with the injured. I favor the hypothesis that the latency-age child's greater awareness of and investment in body image increases the likelihood of linking anxious affect and intrusive memories of the trauma to autonomic and sensory perceptions expressed as physical symptoms.

The manifestations of PTSD during adolescence tend to resemble the adult syndrome (Eth 1989). However, there is one important feature of adolescence that is exaggerated after a traumatic event: the tendency for acting-out behavior. Traumatized teenagers are predisposed to engage in truancy, sexual indiscretion, substance abuse, and delinquency. The use of illicit drugs and alcohol may serve to relieve the dysphoric symptoms of PTSD; self-destructive behavior may be an unconscious effort to expiate guilt. These adolescents adopt a rebellious attitude that seems impervious to limit setting by adults. Some adolescents may embark on a desperate search for a new community in the aftermath of a large-scale disaster. A premature escape into adulthood that is precipitated by trauma is usually doomed to failure, prompting intense feelings of anger, shame, and betrayal. Adolescents can conceive of the effect the trauma will have on their lives. They are sensitive to social stigma and may feel obligated to alter their career and marriage plans accordingly.

School Consultation Technique

The evaluation and treatment of the traumatized child have been the subjects of notable articles and reviews (e.g., Pynoos and Eth 1986; Terr 1987). However, as relevant and important as these topics are, for the purpose of this volume, a public health perspective will take precedence. When a large-scale disaster strikes, the resources for providing individual psychiatric examination and treatment of hundreds or thousands of individual children are uniformly inadequate. What is needed most is a mental health service that can reach the entire population at the time of greatest need. Over the last decade, the Psychological Trauma Center, affiliated with Cedars-Sinai Medical Center in Los Angeles, California, has been perfecting a school-based group consultation program for use in the aftermath of a community-wide trauma. Although the center has been most active in responding to incidents of lethal violence, this program has also proven valuable in responding to earthquakes, fires, and other natural disasters. Our technique serves as a practical strategy when a population of children have been affected by the same event. The goals of this group intervention are to help students and teachers cope more successfully with traumatic stress, to identify those children who are most severely affected and require special attention, and to remedy disruption in school functioning. The school consultation technique is explained through each of its sequential stages (see Table 6–1), and a discussion of its theoretical foundation and clinical application then follows.

Table 6–1. School consultation technique

Preconsultation
1. Identification of incident or need
2. Contact with school principal
3. Preparation on-site

Consultation in class
1. Opening phase
   a. Introduction
   b. Open discussion (fantasy)
   c. Focused discussion (fact)
2. Trauma phase
   a. Free-drawing task
   b. Drawing or story exploration
   c. Reassurance and redirection

3. Closure phase
   a. Recapitulation of fantasy and fact
   b. Sharing of common themes
   c. Return to school activities

Postconsultation
1. Debriefing with school personnel
2. Triage referral
3. Containment and relief

The preconsultation stage of the intervention begins with the recognition that a disaster has occurred. It is safe to assume that all large-scale traumatic events will be immediately reported by the media. Although some communities and school districts have a disaster plan and crisis response team in place, many areas lack adequate preparedness. In such instances, or if the disaster overwhelms available resources, outside assistance is critical. The school principal usually is relieved when a mental health team proactively contacts the school and offers professional services. By deferring mental health responsibility to the crisis team, the principal can devote that much more attention to all the other issues confronting the school in the aftermath of a disaster. The crisis team coordinator discusses the current situation at the school with the principal by telephone. Effective planning depends on information about the nature of the incident, including the extent of damages and the degree of exposure of the students. The presence of other risk factors, such as previous traumatic events, should also be elicited.

Arrangements for the on-site program should be finalized as rapidly as possible. Although a comprehensive consultation would encompass a full range of mental health services for school administrators, support staff, teachers, parents, and families, as detailed by Pynoos and Nader (1988), I focus here only on the classroom consultation itself. Ideally, four consultant therapists would be assigned to each targeted classroom to conduct the 1- to 2-hour session. Therapists from all of the mental health disciplines that work with children are appropriate team members. We have found that child fellows, psychiatry residents, psychology interns, and other clinical trainees are also well suited to be recruited as members of the team. Initially they can observe the more experienced team members as they readily learn to apply their own clinical skills to this particular task. Although we prefer to bring our own art materials (colored markers and large white paper), most schools are equipped to provide an unlimited supply of basic art supplies. The use of the regular classroom prevents logistical confusion in a school that may already be beset by chaos and ensures access to a fixed group of children who are already comfortable expressing themselves in that setting. Consequently, the principal can be reassured that there will be minimal disruption caused by an essentially self-contained intervention.

At the appointed hour, the consultant therapists meet at the school office. The therapists will usually meet briefly with the principal or other school official and outline the plan of services. Each of the targeted classrooms is identified, and any special features that might be relevant to the intervention are discussed. Special education classes and classes for those students who are severely emotionally disturbed may require a larger therapist-student ratio and a slower, more deliberate approach. We prefer to have the classroom teacher present during the session to allay the children's anxieties and to provide the teacher with a therapeutic frame for the children's behavioral and emotional symptoms. Most schools will wish to distribute notices to all parents of the scheduled consultation, thereby permitting them the option of requesting that their child not participate in this activity. In our experience it is the exceptional parent who denies a child the opportunity to partake in a crisis service at school at no fee. However, in those instances, the child can be assigned to another class or to study hall for the hour or two of the consultation.

Following the organizational meeting, the team members enter the classroom, and the consultation with the children begins. During the opening phase of the intervention, each of the team members is introduced by professional title (e.g., "Dr. Eth") while they stand in front of the class. The senior therapist thanks the teacher and asks the children if anyone knows or would like to guess why the team was invited to join the class that day. If one of the team members is a "doctor," a child may suppose that they will have their vision or hearing checked. Other erroneous hypotheses may be offered, until some of the children relate the team's presence to the recent event.

A focus is then established on the disaster or trauma, and the children are encouraged to contribute what they know or have heard about the event and its consequences. Often the children will verbalize their own fearful imagination as if the information was something they had been told by someone else. During the first 10–30 minutes the children are allowed to contribute freely to the discussion as long as they raise their hand and wait to be called on before speaking. Eventually the therapists begin to validate only the information that appears to be accurate, in an effort to correct misunderstanding and contain anxious fantasies. The ability of the consultants to accept openly and calmly the tragic facts is itself an important element of the therapeutic agenda. During this period the team members assess the group's global functioning and note any additional areas of concern that should be explored later in the session.

The children at this point are generally restless and eager to engage in some purposeful activity. The trauma phase commences when the therapists distribute art materials and instruct the children to draw whatever they would like. We assure them that artistic ability is not important and that it is a chance for them to use any color to draw any kind of picture. Most children readily embark on this free-drawing task, and by so doing bind their anxiety and further the process of trauma mastery. In their clinical interview for the recently traumatized child, Pynoos and Eth (1986) also employ a free-drawing technique. This activity allows for the child's imagination to be relieved temporarily from reality and superego constraints and helps counter the detachment and passivity of the posttraumatic state. While the children are busy drawing, the therapists circulate throughout the class, stopping to speak with individual children as they complete their pictures. Not uncommonly children will proceed to create a series of drawings expressing a progression of feelings from superficial and banal to personal and intense.

For those children who have been deeply affected by the disaster, it is assumed that their drawing will contain a reference to the traumatic event. Some children will illustrate the scene of the disaster in exquisite detail; others will draw a picture in which the traumatic association is more obscure. Asking the child to describe the drawing or to make up a story about it may clarify possible connections to the event. Occasionally it may be necessary to remark that although the beautiful scene in the picture is fine, perhaps other things come to mind that can be drawn as well. Not uncommonly the next drawing will reveal more clearly some aspect of the trauma. Of course, some children are not afflicted with intrusive, dysphoric memories or frightening thoughts. Those fortunate students will produce routine art that can be addressed quickly, sparing the child and the therapist from a lengthy and unproductive discussion. The children whose associations to the traumatic event seem to signify conflict, as disclosed by their drawings, stories, or conversation, will have a more extensive therapeutic encounter.

Through the medium of the child's art production, the therapist may be able to explore certain key aspects of the traumatic experience. The therapist can inquire about the extent of the child's exposure to death or destruction. Those children who were eyewitnesses may be expected to retain vivid visual memories accompanied by feelings of anxiety with somatic sensations and perhaps distressing dreams. It can be enormously comforting for the child to have the opportunity to share these symptoms with an adult authority figure. The therapist may wish to reassure the child that these symptoms are the expectable consequences of being the victim of a disaster and that over time their intensity will diminish. It is certainly appropriate to remind the student that fortunately disasters occur only rarely. In cases of violence, the child must contend with issues of human accountability, including the child's own sense of guilt. Most children recognize that assailants are not normal, but may be mentally ill or intoxicated. Especially in inner-city areas, the students will associate the violence with other violent perpetrators they have seen or known. Occasionally a child may reveal that a parent or other relative has been aggressive. Such information may be transmitted to the principal during the debriefing session.

The closure phase of the classroom consultation commences after all of the children have been engaged in a face-to-face encounter. The therapists reassemble together and call the class back to order. The team members recapitulate the information and misinformation gathered about the traumatic event, and add to it descriptions of the typical emotional reactions reported by the students. For example, a common theme of fears and nightmares may be discussed as a normal response to extreme stress. This maneuver provides a further measure of reassurance to the children who may be suffering from that symptom but were too embarrassed to disclose it to a therapist. We also validate the belief that not everyone is alike, so that it is all right to feel differently from one's classmates. It is important to convey to the group that people are available who want to help. We encourage the children to share their concerns with parents, teachers, counselors, and other adults. In some instances a discussion of school safety procedures may serve to protect and provide a concrete set of behaviors that can contain anticipatory anxiety. As the session comes to an end we routinely vocalize our appreciation to the school staff for allowing us to meet with the class, and we compliment the students for their participation. We then redirect their attention to the learning tasks at hand.

Certain modifications of technique are indicated with much younger and older children. Preschool through first-grade classes tend to have more difficulty modulating their excitement and anxiety. These groups tend to need a fuller one-to-one exploration and generally require additional therapist support. High school students may appear less fearful, but they are often highly sensitive to peer pressure and quite reluctant to reveal openly their symptoms. Further, adolescents may resent the intrusion of an outsider into the class and react with hostile guardedness. They also may prove to be surprisingly inhibited artistically and insist on only writing words or simple stick figures on their paper. The therapists must be flexible and willing to accommodate the tenor and demands of the group. However, in our experience, once a few students begin to express themselves in any form, the process usually unfolds without significant resistance.

The postconsultation stage involves a thorough debriefing with the school principal and other interested personnel. This is the team's opportunity to convey an appraisal of how the school, targeted classes, and children are functioning. The principal is given the specific names of children who were identified as needing formal assessment. These are children who may be suffering significant traumatic symptoms either as a result of the disaster or from some other, perhaps unknown, cause. Often the principal will already be aware of these "problem" students. In a situation where the trauma is ongoing, such as the kidnapping of a child who is still missing, follow-up consultations may be scheduled. Not infrequently the principal may suggest a meeting with the teachers or with the school's parent-teacher association (Pynoos and Nader 1988). We will honor those requests and prepare for a session that combines a mixture of didactic material on coping and time for ventilation of feelings. We always depart with the assurance that the school can call us for further advice at any time.

Theoretical Foundation

Our particular technique of group trauma consultation has evolved from a tradition of crisis intervention dating back to the 1940s and Erich Lindemann's (1944) work with the bereaved survivors of Boston's 1942 Coconut Grove nightclub fire. Although the original practice of crisis intervention was developed to assist individuals and families cope with severe stress, the same principles have been applied to work with groups of persons who have been exposed to a common stressor (Ching et al. 1981). It has been well documented that children, like their adult counterparts, will respond symptomatically to a variety of traumatic events, such as a devastating flood (Newman 1976), a major blizzard (Burke et al. 1982), a sniper attack (Pynoos et al. 1987), and the death of a classmate's mother (McDonald 1964). Further, their symptoms may persist for months and years (Burke et al. 1986; Nader et al. 1990).

When a population of children is in crisis, the choice of a site for the intervention is critical. The neighborhood school may be the ideal location. It is generally recognized that schools exert a powerful influence on the child's life (Jellinek 1990), and that children readily discuss their feelings during structured school activities (Bloch et al. 1956). Further, the relative comfort of a familiar environment promotes rapid engagement of the child in the session, and involving the teaching staff can prolong and maximize the effects of the intervention. These considerations are especially important for children living in chaotic homes and socioeconomically disadvantaged neighborhoods. Most importantly, the continuous availability of a large number of target children ensures efficiency and economy.

There are some potential difficulties associated with school-based trauma consultations. In the context of psychotherapy, Nicol (1979) pointed out that confidentiality may be compromised in a school setting. However, the existence of the traumatic incident is usually known throughout the school; participation in group sessions always demands some relaxation of strict therapist-patient secrecy. Another possible problem is that students and teachers may perceive themselves as being "crazy" or mentally ill once they have spoken to a psychiatrist or therapist. Here too, the inclusion of an entire class in the group session minimizes this propensity for adverse labeling. The therapist may feel constrained by an educational social system in which procedures and hierarchical lines of authority abound. Although some limitations do apply, there is the inherent freedom of being an outsider from a different professional background. Finally, it should be acknowledged that there may be obstacles to reimbursement when mental health services are delivered in this fashion. Overall, the balance strongly favors school-based crisis interventions.

Clinical Applications

Several examples of a school-based approach have appeared in the literature (see Table 6–2). For example, two child therapists visited a nearby fourth-grade class 2 weeks after the May 1974 assault on the SLA Headquarters in Los Angeles (Landgarten 1981). The single, art-oriented encounter afforded some relief for the children frightened by that episode of lethal violence. Danto (1983) chronicled his involvement with an elementary school in the wake of the murder of a teacher in her classroom. He recognized that the event traumatized the student witnesses and severely stressed other students, staff, and parents. Although Danto's meetings with school staff and parents were valuable, no attempt was made to reach all of the affected children. In another case, two psychological consultants (one of whom was a parent of a student) accompanied the principal to a classroom for a "show-and-tell" discussion of the funeral of the third-grade teacher (Brooks et al. 1985). None of the children had witnessed the teacher's unexpected death, although they had been deeply affected. The single session permitted the children to share a range of emotions and was viewed positively by staff and parents. Similarly, two therapists entered a private Armenian community school in Los Angeles within a week of the massive earthquake in Soviet Armenia that killed at least 25,000 people in December 1988 (Yacoubian and Hacker 1989). Despite the fact that all of the students were safely living thousands of miles away from the devastation, the group strongly identified with the victims of the earthquake and felt that the catastrophe personally affected their lives. Some even resented not having been a participant in the communal disaster.

Table 6–2.   Examples of school-based interventions

Reference	Incident
Landgarten 1981	Police assault in the neighborhood
Klingman and Eli 1981	Terrorist attack in the neighborhood
Danto 1983	Murder of a teacher in class
Eth et al. 1985a	Murder of a student and parent at home
Eth et al. 1985b	Stabbing of two students at home
Brooks et al. 1985	Death and funeral of a teacher
Eth 1987	Suicidal behavior of a student at school
Pynoos et al. 1987, Nader et al. 1990	Sniper attack on a school playground
Klingman 1987, Klingman et al. 1987	Fatal school bus collision
Kneisel and Richards 1988	Suicide of a teacher
Yacoubian and Hacker 1989	Armenian earthquake for United States students

Israeli Reports

Israeli clinicians have been particularly interested in school-based trauma services. Klingman and Eli (1981) described a crisis intervention after a terrorist attack on a border town. The authors first surveyed the town's schools and documented a high rate of absenteeism, anxiety, poor concentration, and somatic complaints among the students. A consultation team then provided the town's teachers information regarding "disaster-stress syndromes." Consistent with the principles of preventive psychiatry, the crisis was viewed as an opportunity for the children to sharpen their coping skills (Caplan 1970). Over 4 weeks, the authors conducted a series of group sessions designed to reverse emotional disturbances that may have arisen. The sessions began with a focus on ventilation of conscious feelings, later addressing suppressed feelings such as guilt. The process involved verbalization, artwork, guided imagery, and visits to the scene of the attack to achieve emotional catharsis, insight, and conflict resolution.

Klingman (1987) later described a much larger effort in response to a collision of a train with a school bus that resulted in 22 deaths and was witnessed by three other busloads of children. The first task was to prioritize and coordinate the psychological interventions. On the day of the accident, therapists were available to meet with the parents gathered at the school awaiting news of the survivors. The team met with the returning children and their teachers and assisted in the painful process of death notification, an activity associated with considerable stress for both the messenger and the recipient of the news (Eth et al. 1987). The next morning the team identified the child witnesses as a high-risk group, and therapists were assigned to conduct several sessions with each of these classes according to Klingman and Eli's (1981) model. Another target group consisted of children who were related to or very close friends with those who had been killed or injured. All of the teachers were provided with guidance in the use of open discussions in their classes about the tragedy. A "creativity room" was established as a referral site for withdrawn and troubled children. In this room the children were encouraged to express their feelings through drawings, collages, poems, and free writing. A system was organized to visit the children who remained absent from school. Various services were offered to parents, including a telephone hot line, group meetings, and individual and family counseling. This very comprehensive crisis program was predicated on three lessons learned from the Israeli military (Solomon and Benbenishty 1986). First, the intervention was designed to respond rapidly to the school community's horror, grief, and apprehension (immediacy). Second, the activities were school based and involved all of the high-risk children (proximity). Third, the goal was to promote resolution of symptoms so that the school could resume its educational mission (expectancy).

The function of the creativity room is described in greater detail by Klingman et al. (1987). The room was intended to benefit primarily those children who were having difficulty expressing themselves verbally or who were electively mute in the aftermath of the school bus disaster. The children could spend as long as they wished in the creativity room surrounded by art materials and in the presence of an art therapist. Of the approximately 100 collected art productions, about half portrayed the accident. Many also contained written words, often the names of the children who had been killed. A small number of drawings depicted either graves or the image of a dead child. Some of the children drew a series of pictures demonstrating the working through of their grief. In general the art progressed from stiff and stereotyped patterns to more spontaneous and personal drawings. Art is a socially accepted medium of expression that facilitates emotional release through the creation of a permanent product that can later serve as a stimulus for discussion. The authors contended that a single art-oriented session could be a therapeutic and even prophylactic experience. They also noted that the presence of other children in the room further encouraged each youngster to address disaster-related themes.

Psychological Trauma Center

The Psychological Trauma Center has reported examples of its school-based program. In one such consultation we worked with a small, cooperative nursery school after a 4-year-old student and his mother were murdered in their home (Eth et al. 1985a). Separate group sessions were held at the school with the teachers, parents, 4- and 5-year-olds, and 2- and 3-year-olds. We noted that these young children reacted symptomatically to the tragedy and that their usual caretakers (parents and teachers) were unable to respond effectively because of their own grief. Fortunately the affected children proved susceptible to outside therapeutic influence within their familiar school setting. We chose to employ modeling clay with the youngest children because of their difficulty using conventional markers and paper. We contend that the overriding benefit with these preschoolers derived not from the provision of factual information but from the emotional exchange between consultant and child. Immediate and (as follow-up contact indicated) lasting relief of anxiety was generated by the reassuring presence of adults who gave testimony to the belief that terrible events could be openly discussed and mastered. The preventative aspect of the consultation arose from the affective communication, which is at the heart of any therapeutic activity and which repairs the child's sense of the presence of a protective shield offered by trusted adults.

We have also reported a consultation to a large, public elementary school in the aftermath of an episode of family violence that resulted in injury to two brothers enrolled in the school (Eth et al. 1985b). Although the incident was not witnessed by the pupils, the intrusion of violence into the school community precipitated anxiety in the students and teachers, prompting disturbing behaviors and disrupting the educational process. The injured boys were visited by the psychiatric liaison to the pediatric ward while they were hospitalized at the county medical center. Contact was then made with the principal of their elementary school, who was extremely receptive to the offer of a violence-focused consultation. The principal assisted the trauma team in identifying and collecting the children considered most likely to be affected by the widely publicized incident. These groups included the kindergarten and second-grade classmates of the two injured boys and all of those students who routinely rode the school bus with them. Separate sessions were held with the two classes attended by the boys and with groups of 20 bus mates assembled by grade level (kindergarten, first and second grade, third and fourth grade, and fifth and sixth grade).

The sessions began with introductions by the team and then proceeded directly to an elicitation of the children's fantasies about what had occurred and why. The children seemed eager to share what they had heard and imagined, although not all of the information offered was accurate. The team calmly disclosed the truth about the violence to dispel the wild rumors and to refocus the group on the actual event. The therapists sought to demonstrate that there are adults who will tolerate hearing and talking openly about violence, despite any prohibition against discussion the children may have faced. The silence enforced by well-meaning but misguided parents and teachers may transmit the unintended message that the subject is too frightening or overwhelming ever to mention aloud, thereby reinforcing the children's anxiety (Lister 1982). Paper and colored markers were distributed, and all of the children were instructed to draw whatever they liked. This structured activity decreased the children's restlessness, while providing the opportunity for them to express themselves creatively.

While the children were engaged in their free-drawing task, the therapists circulated throughout the group. In face-to-face interactions, the children were questioned about their artwork, with special attention given to aggressive themes, identifications, and conspicuous fears, depression, or denial. Several students commented on tensions in their own homes and their personal concerns about family violence. The projective use of an art technique affords the therapist a readily accessible medium for appropriate clarifications and interpretations. Often a child will construct a series of drawings illustrating the progression of the therapeutic interaction. Although the art products from the groups displayed developmental differences, several themes recurred. Many children drew the scene of violence, often with extreme exaggeration. Some children chose to depict incidents of violence that they had witnessed and had not previously revealed. One child drew a camper truck crashing into a car and killing all of the passengers. He then disclosed that he was in an accident on the highway some months earlier that he thought he had forgotten, but that had begun to trouble him greatly since his friend was injured. The concept of family violence was upsetting, especially to the younger children, who preferred to replace the human perpetrator with ferocious animals or horrible witches. Depressive elements appeared as pictures of cemeteries and funerals. Other children dwelled on religious images in an effort to find comfort and security in an out-of-control society.

The session entered a closing phase with the children reassembling to summarize the discussions. The team recapitulated the reality of the violent event in the framework of the therapeutic consultation. Importantly, the therapists explored what it would be like for the injured boys to return to school and how each child might facilitate the process. One child proudly told the group that he had given toys to the boys because he had been so upset about them. The focus was then directed to the learning tasks that had been interfered with by the violent episode and its aftermath. On that note, the teams left the classroom and debriefed the principal, relaying the names of the students who appeared to require follow-up attention. Because of the widespread interest in the consultation, I was invited to attend the next faculty meeting. The consultation methodology was reviewed and some of the artwork was displayed. The teachers responded by indicating that the teams had achieved their goals of relieving anxiety in the affected students, easing the boys' return to school, and lifting the responsibility from the teachers to discuss the distressing topic of family violence. Almost without exception, the children who had been in the sessions had performed well the rest of the day. One teacher wondered whether innocent children should be exposed to the details of such violence. Her colleagues quickly reassured her that the children in their school were already quite knowledgeable about the threat of violence. Subsequent contact with the school confirmed the impression of a successful therapeutic consultation.

Suicide

Each traumatic event has its own characteristic effects on victims and witnesses. A sudden incident of self-destructive behavior by a student will, in most instances, precipitate in the school community reactions similar to those arising from other forms of human-induced violence. Children are both frightened and fascinated by suicidal acts. Certainly students as young as sixth graders can appreciate the meaning of taking one's own life (Eth et al. 1984). It is an immediate source of anxiety to know someone who has made a suicide attempt. When death results from the act, the children and school staff are also forced to contend with feelings of sadness and grief. Not uncommonly, a child's association leads to the personal loss of a beloved family member. Occasionally, children express guilt over a perceived failure to have intervened to save their friend's life.

Fortunately, in our experience, the majority of children faced with a suicidal crisis in a school will respond to our group consultation with increased mastery of anxiety and sadness, and as a class with an increased sense of cohesion and purpose. In fact, we have not found it necessary to modify our usual technique, although the content will reflect suicidal themes (Eth 1987). There is reason to be concerned that the awareness of a suicide may itself promote suicidal behavior in certain susceptible adolescents as a contagion effect (Phillips and Carstensen 1986). However, the finding that children will openly report suicidal ideation during the consultation holds promise that the early identification of these otherwise silent students may reduce the likelihood of further suicidal behavior.

Kneisel and Richards (1988) described a series of classroom discussions they conducted after a particularly horrifying suicide by a fifth- and sixth-grade teacher. These authors were sensitive to the danger of imitation behavior, but felt that the opportunity to reduce confusion, secrecy, and rumors surrounding a suicide would lead to decreased anxiety, depression, and distrust within the school community and thereby lessen the risk of additional suicidal acts. The authors employed an educational approach, emphasizing the transmission of information about the suicide in a nonjudgmental and caring question-and-answer format. Although lacking formal outcome data, the authors believe that their response contributed to the healing process and served to minimize mental health difficulties that would have been expected to arise after a teacher's suicide.

Disaster at a School

When major violence directly involves the school itself, the emotional consequences for the students and staff are widespread. Pynoos et al. (1987) studied a Los Angeles elementary school after a fatal sniper attack on the playground. Within days of the shooting, the investigators interviewed 159 children exposed in varying degrees to this isolated episode of life-threatening violence. Their findings show a clear dose-response relationship between proximity to the violence and symptomatology. The symptom score for the children under direct fire was twice as great as that for those children who were already walking home and four times that of the youngsters who were not in school on the day of the attack. At least 80% of the severely exposed children described the immediate onset of a full range of posttraumatic symptoms, regardless of age, sex, or ethnicity. The children who were not in direct danger rarely demonstrated acute PTSD unless other situational risk factors were also present. Feelings of guilt and knowledge of the deceased victim were both correlated with higher symptom scores.

The situation of an entire school becoming dysfunctional in the aftermath of campus violence is reminiscent of Kai Erikson's (1976) description of the "loss of communality" afflicting the town of Buffalo Creek, West Virginia, after a catastrophic flood in February 1972. The value of a group intervention is thereby expanded, as the technique has the effect of repairing the collective "trauma membrane" (Lindy et al. 1983), as well as relieving individuals' symptoms of anxiety. In a school where the majority of children have been affected by disaster, every classroom deserves a consultation, which was done at the school site of the sniper attack. Nonetheless, a 14-month follow-up assessment of 100 of the original 159 children surveyed found reduction but not eradication of traumatic symptoms, especially in the children who had been most seriously affected (Nader et al. 1990). As the study suggests, a school exposed to human-induced or natural disaster needs both a crisis-oriented intervention and a follow-up treatment program for the traumatized children who remain symptomatic.

Conclusion

Primary prevention of the morbid responses to traumatic life events would require the eradication of natural disasters and human-induced violence. Sadly, any such effort is doomed to failure. Although the precise time and location of the next earthquake, hurricane, or sniper attack is unknown, it is virtually certain that these calamities will befall us. However, despite the inevitability of trauma, strategies may be implemented to minimize the resulting distress and disability arising in susceptible children. In this chapter I have reviewed the phenomenology of posttraumatic syndromes, and I have presented a model classroom intervention. This therapeutic technique holds promise of being an economical and effective community response in the aftermath of disaster. It is imperative that our political and educational leaders provide every child at risk the benefits of a mental health service at the time of greatest need. Clinicians have the means to meet this need; we only await the opportunity to act.

References

American Psychiatric Association: Diagnostic and Statistical Manual of Mental Disorders, 3rd Edition, Revised. Washington, DC, American Psychiatric Association, 1987

Bloch DA, Silber E, Perry SE: Some factors in the emotional reactions of children to disaster. Am J Psychiatry 113:416–422, 1956

Brooks B, Silverman G, Hass RG: When a teacher dies: a school-based intervention with latency children. Am J Orthopsychiatry 55:405–410, 1985

Burke JD, Borus JF, Burns BJ, et al: Some factors in the emotional reaction of children to disaster. Am J Psychiatry 139:1010–1014, 1982

Burke JD, Moccia P, Borus JF, et al: Emotional distress in fifth-grade children ten months after a natural disaster. J Am Acad Child Psychiatry 25:536–541, 1986

Caplan G: The Theory and Practice of Mental Health Consultation. New York, Basic Books, 1970

Ching JWJ, Gordon R, O'Mahoney MT: Crisis intervention following severe psychological trauma in late pregnancy. Hosp Community Psychiatry 32:53–56, 1981

Danto BL: A man came and killed our teacher, in The Child and Death. Edited by Schowalter JE, Patterson PR, Tallmer M, et al. New York, Columbia University Press, 1983, pp 49–74

Erikson KT: Loss of communality at Buffalo Creek. Am J Psychiatry 133:302–305, 1976

Eth S: School consultation following suicidal behavior, in Proceedings of the Twentieth Annual Conference of the American Association of Suicidology. Edited by Yufit RI. San Francisco, CA, American Association of Suicidology, 1987, pp 390–391

Eth S: The adolescent witness to homicide, in Juvenile Homicide. Edited by Benedek EP, Cornell DG. Washington, DC, American Psychiatric Press, 1989, pp 86–113

Eth S: Post-traumatic stress disorder in childhood, in Handbook of Child and Adult Psychopathology. Edited by Hersen M, Last CG. New York, Pergamon, 1990, pp 263–274

Eth S, Pynoos RS: Developmental perspective on psychic trauma in childhood, in Trauma and Its Wake. Edited by Figley CR. New York, Brunner/Mazel, 1985, pp 36–52

Eth S, Pynoos RS, Carlson GA: An unusual case of self-inflicted death in childhood. Suicide Life Threat Behav 14:157–165, 1984

Eth S, Silverstein S, Pynoos RS: Mental health consultation to a preschool following the murder of a mother and child. Hosp Community Psychiatry 36:73–76, 1985a

Eth S, Arroyo W, Silverstein S: A psychiatric crisis team response to violence in elementary schools, in Expanding Mental Health Interventions in Schools. Edited by Berkovitz IH, Seliger JS. Dubuque, IA, Kendall/Hunt, 1985b, pp 55–62

Eth S, Baron D, Pynoos RS: Death notification. Bull Am Acad Psychiatry Law 15:275–281, 1987

Eth S, Randolph ET, Brown JA: Post-traumatic stress disorder, in Modern Perspectives in the Psychiatry of the Neuroses. Edited by Howells JG. New York, Brunner/Mazel, 1989, pp 210–234

Jellinek MS: School consultation: evolving issues. J Am Acad Child Adolesc Psychiatry 29:311–314, 1990

Kinston W, Rosser R: Disaster: effects on mental and physical state. J Psychosom Res 18:437–456, 1974

Klingman A: A school-based emergency crisis intervention in a mass school disaster. Professional Psychology 18:604–612, 1987

Klingman A, Eli ZE: A school community in disaster: primary and secondary prevention in situational crisis. Professional Psychology 12:523–533, 1981

Klingman A, Koenigsfeld E, Markman D: Art activity with children following disaster. Arts Psychotherapy 14:153–166, 1987

Kneisel PJ, Richards GP: Crisis intervention after the suicide of a teacher. Professional Psychology 19:165–169, 1988

Landgarten HB: Clinical Art Therapy. New York, Brunner/Mazel, 1981

Lindemann E: Symptomatology and management of acute grief. Am J Psychiatry 101:141–148, 1944

Lindy JD, Green BL, Grace M, et al: Psychotherapy with survivors of the Beverly Hills Supper Club fire. Am J Psychother 37:593–610, 1983

Lister ED: Forced silence: a neglected dimension of trauma. Am J Psychiatry 139:867–872, 1982

McDonald M: Children's reactions to the death of a mother. Psychoanal Stud Child 19:558–376, 1964

Nader K, Pynoos RS, Fairbanks L, et al: Children's PTSD reactions one year after a sniper attack at their school. Am J Psychiatry 147:1526–1530, 1990

Newman J: Children of disaster: clinical observation at Buffalo Creek. Am J Psychiatry 133:306–312, 1976

Nicol AR: Psychotherapy and the school. J Child Psychol Psychiatry 20:81–86, 1979

Phillips D, Carstensen L: Clustering of teenage suicides after television news stories about suicide. N Engl J Med 315:685–689, 1986

Pynoos RS, Eth S: Witness to violence: the child interview. J Am Acad Child Psychiatry 25:306–319, 1986

Pynoos RS, Nader K: Psychological first aid and treatment approach to children exposed to community violence: research implications. Journal of Traumatic Stress 1:445–473, 1988

Pynoos RS, Frederick C, Nader K, et al: Life threat and posttraumatic stress in school-age children. Arch Gen Psychiatry 144:1057–1063, 1987

Solomon Z, Benbenishty R: The role of proximity, immediacy, and expectancy in frontline treatment of combat stress reaction among Israelis in the Lebanon War. Am J Psychiatry 143:613–617, 1986

Terr LC: Childhood psychic trauma, in Basic Handbook of Child Psychiatry, Vol 5. Edited by Noshpitz JD. New York, Basic Books, 1987, pp 262–272

Terr LC: What happens to early memories of trauma? J Am Acad Child Adolesc Psychiatry 27:96–104, 1988

Terr LC: Childhood traumas: an outline and overview. Am J Psychiatry 148:10–20, 1991

Turkel SB, Eth S: Psychopathological responses to stress: adjustment disorder and post-traumatic stress disorder in children and adolescents, in Childhood Stress. Edited by Arnold LE. New York, Wiley, 1990, pp 51–71

Yacoubian VV, Hacker FJ: Reactions to disaster at a distance. Bull Menninger Clin 53:331–339, 1989

Chapter 7

Interacting With the Media After Trauma in the Community

Harvey L. Ruben, M.D., M.P.H.

*T*hroughout this volume, we have been looking at various disasters and the consequences they have for those who are affected directly and indirectly in the surrounding community. The main way that we learn about these disasters and their impact on the community is through the media. The media are a very powerful tool for public information and education. Television, in particular, through the use of visual imagery, has the greatest impact. By 1987, 98% of all the homes in the United States had at least one television set, and 68% had more than one television set. The average home had the television set on for approximately 7 hours a day. Of the general public, 66% stated that they used television to obtain most of their news, and 50% believed that television was the most reliable source of news (Broadcasting and Cable Yearbook 1989).

General Principles

Especially in the midst of a community disaster, people are more dependent on the media for gaining information. No matter what has happened, they are hungry for news: What is the extent of the disaster? How many people have been affected? What public services are available or have been lost? What mechanisms for support and therapeutic services are in place? Because community disasters are so intrinsically stressful, appropriate and adequate information is crucial to help alleviate the stress and trauma.

In the case of Hurricane Hugo in September 1989, in which prolonged, major power outages occurred, the only link to the outside world for many was a portable radio or, if they were lucky, a battery-operated television set. On my nationally syndicated radio call-in show for several weeks after Hurricane Hugo, I had callers from the Charleston, South Carolina, area who said they were without power and were using the radio and telephone as their link to the outside world as they attempted to reconstruct their lives.

In many disasters, people use the full range of print and electronic media programming for useful information on the nature and extent of the disaster through news reports. They also rely on television and radio talk shows and call-in programs for an analysis of the situation and a broader base of data to help them determine how to proceed. When a disaster occurs, an entire community of tens of thousands of people or even more may be traumatized by the event. Obviously, our traditional approaches of individual or small-group therapy are totally insufficient to deal with the magnitude of the community disturbance, and the media may be used to facilitate the emotional working through of the disaster by the entire community.

Mental health professionals working at disaster sites have developed the techniques of large-group "debriefings" to help a greater number of involved individuals cope with trauma. During the debriefing meetings, mental health workers will talk to those affected about the nature of the event and what the involved individuals may be feeling. This is followed by a question-and-answer session to allow people to deal with their own particular issues. The goals of these large-group sessions include reassuring the victims of the normalcy of their feelings, providing a way of identifying and naming their emotions and responses, providing instructions in various self-help techniques, and alerting victims to warning signs that would indicate the need for further treatment. Such techniques have been well developed and utilized by a number of different authors of various chapters in this volume, where they are described in more detail. At times, however, the extent of the disaster is so great and the impact so overwhelming that these person-to-person techniques are inadequate. In such circumstances, the media offer a powerful means to debrief a large population. In essence, the spokesperson then acts as a "mass"-group psychotherapist by using the same debriefing model on radio or television to achieve the goals mentioned above (Austin, Chapter 3, this volume).

After a disaster, both the print and the electronic media are eager to interview mental health professionals concerning the impact of the trauma. Utilizing the techniques used in the group debriefing model, the mental health professional is able to help a large number of involved community members, while also teaching the public about mental health treatment from a positive public relations perspective. There are several potential pitfalls that require the careful attention of the mental health professional involved in such media work. Reporters often ask how people are reacting, and one must comment on the nature and the degree of responses, so that a listener will not tune out because he or she does not identify with the example being presented. Additionally, when reporters ask about available mental health services, as discussed above, one should be prepared to relay that information adequately without creating unrealistic expectations. Given the importance of the media for disseminating this critical information, it is essential that those mental health professionals who interact with the media be effective spokespersons who can give reports and advice in a way that is helpful to the public.

The mental health treatment programs responding directly to the disaster should have one or more individuals who are trained to act as spokespersons. They must have as much information as possible about all aspects of the disaster, its effect, the number of people who have been involved, the likely results for victims, and the local resources available to help deal with the trauma.

The spokesperson should give information only about which he or she is certain. If there are areas of uncertainty, this should be clearly stated. One should never attempt to guess without clearly stating that the opinion is based on an estimate rather than on fact. One should be as calm and reassuring as possible, while giving as much information as is available. If the information is negative, the spokesperson should be honest and direct while stating the adverse implications. At the same time one should attempt to stress whatever is positive about the situation or what help is at hand. It is important not to overstate, nor to evade an issue or question, but rather to declare simply that one does not have the information as of yet, but will obtain it and report back as soon as possible.

Because people are very upset after community disasters, the presence of helping resources is critical. Therefore, as soon as possible, a spokesperson should present to the media all available information about the nature, location, and availability of various support services. If at the time of initial contact with the media such information is not available, it should be clearly stated that helping resources are being developed and will be reported to the media in the near future. Specifically, in situations where such information is not available or disaster response teams have yet to be developed, the media can be helpful by identifying those who are in need of help and also those mental health professionals who are in the area who could volunteer to lend a hand. The media can be used to set up a hot line or a central office where those who need help can call and to develop a cadre of workers who have identified themselves and will come to the office.

If at all possible, those who become spokespersons should have had some experience in dealing with the media. However, since this is not always possible, it is important that the spokespersons understand the needs of the reporters with whom they are interacting. I discuss this in greater detail below in relation to each type of print or electronic media outlet. In general, however, the spokesperson must keep in mind that the reporters need to get the news as quickly as possible, because they are always working on an imminent deadline. Under the pressure of obtaining timely information, the potential for misunderstanding exists. Therefore, the spokesperson must be certain that he or she fully understands the reporter's questions and that the reporter fully understands the response. It is acceptable to ask the reporter to repeat the question or to rephrase one's own answer to emphasize some aspect and to ensure that the reporter clearly understands the response.

The American Psychiatric Association's "Guidelines for the Psychiatrist Working With the Communications Media" (1977) contains important pointers for those who become speakers to the media. Since mental health professionals frequently appear on call-in shows giving advice, it is essential to clarify that advice is not treatment. When a person calls in and asks for advice, an appropriate response (in addition to giving advice) is to refer the person for evaluation and treatment, in person, at a local mental health facility. The caveat should be given that advice is not and cannot be expected to be a substitute for evaluation and, if necessary, treatment.

Similarly, the issue of confidentiality is critical when the mental health professional is involved with the media. Psychiatrists should not cite their own cases, even in a composite or fictionalized way, because the listeners or viewers may not understand this and may believe the psychiatrist is talking about his or her patient on the air. If a mental health professional is unsure of an answer, this fact should be clearly stated and the professional should make no comment or should promise to find the answer and return with the appropriate information in the near future. The spokesperson should clarify whom he or she is representing, such as a hospital or the local psychiatric or medical society. If the person is not representing any organized group, this also should be clearly stated.

In dealing with reporters in the print or the electronic media, it is wise to give short, clear, concise answers. If the spokesperson is not well versed in a particular area and does not feel competent to answer, then the reporter should be referred to an expert in that area, rather than the spokesperson hazarding a guess or making an inaccurate statement. It is very important that mental health professionals not comment on particular individuals involved in the news and especially that no one attempt to diagnose a public figure. To do so would be unethical for a number of reasons. Certainly, to make a diagnosis without evaluating a person is inappropriate; if the person has been evaluated, then confidentiality would prevent the mental health professional from commenting.

At times, perhaps because of the pressures under which he or she is operating, the reporter may seem curt, argumentative, or impatient with the spokesperson. In such circumstances, the spokesperson must remain calm and not become angry, but rather be rational, direct, and to the point. If the reporter is directly hostile, the best approach is to use humility, or perhaps humor, if possible. The spokesperson may ask the reporter to repeat, clarify, or expand his or her question to understand better the reasons for the hostility.

Dealing With Specific Types of Media

The above general principles apply to all interactions with the media in the immediate postdisaster period and thereafter. To help the identified spokespersons better interact with the media, I now turn to the different types of media and how best to deal with reporters based on an understanding of their particular needs and format.

Television

Other than in the circumstances where there have been major power outages, the most likely venues for presenting information about a disaster will be television and radio. Because television gives a visual image along with the sound and thereby draws the audience into the scene, most people will turn to television, if it is available, to learn about the disaster. They know that there will be visuals to demonstrate the extent of the disaster. Because television dramatizes and creates so much interest on the part of the viewers, it captures the audience, who are less likely to engage in other activities while watching.

Television is an expensive medium and requires a great deal of preparation (much more than a radio broadcast) to plan and execute a program. News program personnel are most likely to consult mental health professionals during the early phases of the disaster. Television news is slower paced than radio because the viewer must register both the visual and the auditory aspect of the program. However, most news stories are only given 40–90 seconds, with as little as 15–20 seconds for an interview.

If the mental health professional is going to be a guest on a television talk show, there will be much more time both for the interview and, as a rule, for preparation. It is helpful for the mental health professional to be familiar with the television studio if at all possible before going in for an interview or an appearance. If this is not possible, it is acceptable to ask questions about how things are going to occur and what is expected after arriving at the studio. If one is being interviewed at his or her own office or at some other scene, it is also appropriate to ask questions and understand fully how things will be proceeding to help put oneself at ease.

The spokesperson should concentrate on the reporter or the talk show host, attending carefully to the questions and remaining undistracted by elements of production, audiences, or background events. One should always look at the host or the reporter and never look into the camera unless instructed to do so. The monitor should not be looked at, in attempts to "watch the show," because this invariably will result in a picture of the spokesperson looking off into space seemingly uninvolved with what is transpiring. Television audiences are impressed by physical appearance. Therefore, the spokesperson must appear professional both in demeanor and in dress. Clothing worn should be conservative and appear professional, without much jewelry or other items of clothing that could distract the audience. The spokesperson should establish his or her academic credentials; in the case of psychiatrists, the interviewer should understand that this connotes an M.D.

Given the short length of time for any television news spot, brevity is critical. Although an interview may last 30 minutes for a piece that will appear on the evening news, it will be edited to a very short, fast segment to fit the requirements of the program. Therefore, one should speak in brief, concise, declarative sentences that state a viewpoint as clearly as possible. Interesting and simple language should be used, as this will make it easier to edit and pick out appropriate segments of the interview. In such a brief interview, it is possible to make only one or two main points. These are called in media terms "SOCO" statements: Single Overriding Communications Objectives. One should plan ahead of time the one or two SOCO statements that should be made. These should be mentally rehearsed so that they will be included in the interview. This is the information that is most critical for the audience to know.

The same principles should be followed for interviews conducted live on-air. Again, the spokesperson should remember to look directly at the interviewer and not at the camera or the monitors. One should attempt to be as relaxed and informal as possible, while maintaining a sense of professional stature. This allows the audience to identify with the professional and to understand the intended message. If negative questions are anticipated, one should prepare responses tentatively ahead of time and focus on positive points, if at all possible. The spokesperson should be sincere and tell the truth about the particular situation, while attempting to end on a positive note. One should try to answer all questions in one sentence that will, for the most part, be a self-contained message.

If the spokesperson is appearing on a television talk show, more time will be allowed, and the spokesperson should be prepared to talk in more depth about the material and the topic. One should arrive at the studio early and understand ahead of time who the audience is, how the show is formatted, and what can be expected. It makes good sense to attempt to watch the show before appearing to have a better sense of how things will go. Often some powder or other makeup will be applied before the show. One should sit upright in a chair with legs together or crossed toward the interviewer so the camera does not show the bottom of the shoes. Men should wear over-the-calf socks. Gestures may be made freely, but movements should be kept close to the body, and nervous gestures should be avoided. Although the host will often give the lead when to speak, the spokesperson should not be afraid to interject a pertinent point when it is appropriate. Although it is helpful to attempt to relax and enjoy the interview, it is also important to remember that one has something valuable and newsworthy to share with the audience. It is important to make points clearly for this reason. For further discussion of aspects of television interviews, the reader is referred to *Speaking Out for Psychiatry* (Group for the Advancement of Psychiatry 1981) and *How to Speak TV* (Jones 1983).

Radio

Depending on the type of disaster, radio may be equally important or perhaps even more important than television to transmit information to the community. Unlike television, which requires equipment and a crew, radio requires only a reporter with a tape recorder or a telephone. There are times when the radio reporter may be the first on the scene or the first to interview the mental health professional with a late-breaking story. In instances of power outages, radio may be the sole source of news for the involved community.

Unless the spokesperson is dealing with a radio special about a particular disaster (in which case the spokesperson will have a fair amount of time to discuss the disaster and its implications in depth), radio news, like television, will usually limit responses to 10–20 seconds in an interview. Therefore, the principles outlined above in relation to television news interviews also pertain. Simple, direct, concise answers that are self-contained and perhaps 20 seconds in length will be most easily used. As with television, SOCO statements that clearly communicate main points to the audience should be used. Unlike television, radio is a personal medium that duplicates the one-to-one situation between the speaker and the listener. The auditory stimulus alone holds the listener's interest. Therefore, it is important that what is said is interesting and stimulating, for if the listener's mind wanders, the message is lost. Given that all the radio reporter needs is a tape recorder, it is possible for news interviews to be taped over the telephone. Thus, again, it is critically important that the spokesperson's responses be short and concise and have an impact, making the point and grabbing the listener's attention. Although an interview may last 15 minutes, it is likely that significantly less than a minute will actually air; SOCO statements must be woven into answers if the interview is to be successful. Unlike television, on radio the spokesperson must rely on tone of voice to emphasize key points in answering questions, since what is said and how it is said will create a mental image for the listener.

As with television, it is important to arrive at the studio for a live show at least 15 minutes early and to be certain to ask whatever questions and get whatever information is needed to understand who the audience is, who the potential callers might be, or who the other guests are. Listening to the show ahead of time is always very useful for the spokesperson. As with any news or talk show on television or radio, it is always best to be humble and respectful of the interviewer or host and the callers. Especially if a caller becomes aggressive or hostile, it is important for the professional to maintain professional bearing, not to become irritable, and to answer in an honest and direct fashion. The spokesperson does not need to be concerned about crank calls, because these can be edited or deleted by the engineer without difficulty. One should not let the caller or the host be intimidating; rather the spokesperson should state answers in a positive way, acknowledging that the caller may have a different opinion. Especially when answering questions on a call-in show for those who have suffered trauma in a disaster, the spokesperson should not attempt to diagnose or provide treatment. Rather, the spokesperson should give information and advice on how to understand the nature of the problem and where to go for in-person evaluation and treatment.

Print Media: Newspapers and Magazines

Newspapers and magazines are the oldest form of mass media in the United States and will certainly be actively involved in reporting community disasters. Newspapers, of course, will be under the greatest pressure to get the news out quickly and to give as much in-depth information as possible. Because the reporter is under time pressure, it is imperative for the spokesperson to be able to reply immediately or in the near future to meet the news deadline. Therefore, when the reporter calls, if the spokesperson cannot respond immediately, he or she should find out when the reporter's deadline is. If an interview cannot be given within that time frame, an attempt should be made to locate another spokesperson who will be able to comply with the deadline.

Unlike the electronic media, the print reporter will be taking notes or recording the interview (with permission) to provide accurate quotes and save all appropriate information. There is rarely time in a newspaper article to check with the reporter after the article is written for the accuracy of quotes. Therefore, it is important for the spokesperson to state points clearly and even reemphasize the points in a direct, concise manner to make sure that the reporter has understood clearly.

As in other forms of mass media, space is limited, but unlike the electronic media, newspaper and magazine articles can be reread. Therefore, statements must be direct and to the point and clearly convey the intent of the message. Newspaper reporters often want to quote or cite several sources; if it is possible to identify another appropriate spokesperson for the reporter, this may be useful. Likewise, if there is controversy concerning a particular topic, it is useful to point this out to the reporter and to comment on the opposing views so that when the reporter seeks another viewpoint, one's own position will be known.

Unlike the daily news, articles in the newspaper's feature section and magazine articles have a much longer lead time. Reporters will do in-depth research on the stories they are reporting. Therefore, when a reporter calls for one of these articles, the spokesperson has much more time to contemplate responses and, if necessary, to gather information. One should clarify with the reporter that this is a newspaper feature story or a magazine article and find out when the reporter's deadline is. Then either before or after the interview, the spokesperson has the ability to gather more information so that a much more detailed interview can be given than for a news story.

News story interviews are often carried out over the telephone; feature article and magazine interviews usually are conducted face to face. These writers will usually be looking for as much anecdotal information as possible. Feature stories and magazine articles are often built around personalities, good quotes, and interesting anecdotes, in addition to unusual information and solid facts. Since the spokesperson is the expert for the reporter, and since there is much more time, it is not unreasonable to ask a reporter to call back and read portions of the story to ensure the accuracy of quotations. No statements should be made "off the record" unless one is prepared to see them in print.

Many magazines will accept articles written by nonprofessional writers who are spokespersons for various organizations. It is possible to generate a story about a particular event, such as how one's group or organization responded to a disaster, what the effects on the victims were, and how professionals helped deal with the situation. This is another useful way to educate the public and the community at large about the effects of the community disaster and what can be expected in the future.

Conclusion

The media figure prominently in every disaster. It is through the print and the electronic media that the public and the involved community first learn about the extent of the disaster, what the likely consequences will be, how extensive the disruption to community life has been, and what resources are available to help people cope with this disaster.

In addition to the involved community, people throughout the rest of the country will be learning about these various aspects of the disaster from the print and the electronic media. As mental health professionals, we are involved not only in immediate response to the disaster to help the victims and their families, but we also have an educative responsibility for the rest of the community and the public at large. We must have appropriate spokespersons, either previously identified or identified immediately at the time of the disaster, who can represent this information to the print and the electronic media. Ideally each organization should develop a disaster plan that includes spokesperson training for those who will be dealing with the media at the time of the disaster. If such training cannot be carried out prospectively, then on-the-job training and orientation for those mental health professionals who will be identified as spokespersons by hospital or professional society media relations staff will at least allow the spokespersons to function in an appropriate way.

For the uninitiated, dealing with the media is inevitably anxiety provoking. However, with some careful preparation and with the information contained in this chapter, anyone who will be a media spokesperson should be able to do so adequately. With the additional help of public relations professionals from local hospitals or professional societies, the spokesperson should be able to do a very credible job. Although this activity is not usually seen as a part of the functioning of most mental health professionals, when a disaster places such inordinate demands on all members of the community, it is within the scope of that professional's job to respond to the media; such communication serves to enhance and improve the well-being of the entire community.

References

American Psychiatric Association: Guidelines for the psychiatrist working with the communications media (official actions). Am J Psychiatry 134:609–611, 1977

Broadcasting and Cable Year Book, New York, 1989, p A3

Group for the Advancement of Psychiatry: Speaking Out for Psychiatry: A Handbook for Involvement with the Mass Media (Report No 124). New York, Brunner/Mazel, 1981

Jones C: How to Speak TV: A Self Defense Manual When You Are in the News. Miami, FL, Kirkan & Co, 1983

Case Studies in Community Disaster Response

Chapter 8

The 1989 San Francisco Bay Area Earthquake

Mel Blaustein, M.D.,
Etta C. Bryant, M.D., Alan R. Cole, M.D.,
Lynda Frattaroli, M.S.W., John R. Gillette, M.D.,
Joyce C. Jarvis, M.P.A., Lynn E. Ponton, M.D.

*T*he year before the San Francisco Bay Area Loma Prieta earthquake, the U.S. Geological Survey had identified six California fault segments that were likely to sustain an earthquake in the period from 1988 to 2018 of Richter scale magnitude 6.5 or greater (Plakker and Galloway 1989). Two earthquakes measuring 5.1 and 5.2 in fact shook the Loma Prieta region 2 and 15 months before, respectively, the earthquake of 1989. Public advisories followed these events. Seismologists, largely unheard outside of geologic circles, continued to point out that the stress relieved by the 1906 quake had been building up again to failure level and that only two major quakes had occurred in the ensuing 83 years to defuse the pressure.

The 1989 San Francisco Bay Area Earthquake

No one gave these warnings much heed at the start of Game 3 of the World Series on the evening of October 17, 1989, at San Francisco's Candlestick Park. As ticket holders took their seats and home viewers turned on their televisions, 60 miles southeast of the stadium the North American and Pacific plates were pulling apart on the San Andreas Fault to unleash a 7.1 magnitude earthquake. The area's general good fortune was not entirely inoperative—the epicenter of the earthquake occurred at "probably the most desolate of all regions in Northern California," according to the U.S. Geological Survey (Lindh 1990). Most children were safely out of school, and businesses had closed for the day.

Nonetheless, 67 died, and 3,700 were injured. Of those who died, 42 were crushed under one section of the Nimitz freeway in Oakland. One motorist on the freeway described it as follows:

> It was like a big, giant, long ocean wave, and behind each wave a portion of the freeway collapsed. . . . I just started crying. There was nothing I could do. I could hear a few moans and groans, but I couldn't tell where they were coming from. ("Reaction of the Public" 1989, p. A6)

The earthquake was very selective, targeting mainly parts of San Francisco, Santa Cruz, Oakland, and Watsonville. In all, 1,000 homes were destroyed, and 2,300 were damaged. San Francisco and Oakland each lost nearly 1,000 low-rent units, exacerbating the existing housing shortages and unemployment in these cities. A total of 12,000 persons were left homeless. Repair estimates ranged from $5.9 to $7.0 billion, making the Loma Prieta earthquake one of the most expensive of all natural disasters in American history.

The acute impact stage of the earthquake was followed in the next 6 months by more than 5,000 aftershocks, which kept the affected community at a high pitch of anxiety. Compounding the recovery stage for many was the "second disaster" of bureaucratic snags delaying relocation and rebuilding. A poignant letter to the editor of the *San Jose Mercury News* (Williamson 1990, p. 1A) on the anniversary of the earthquake reflects this:

> Yes my life has changed since October 17, 1989. . . . I am heartbroken. I was thrown down in my backyard and lay watching my beautiful home twisting, writhing, actually moving away from me. When the quake subsided, everything that I had cherished for more than forty years was gone. It's now 11 months since the quake and I have had to cope with councils, commissions, committees, history buffs, and demolition delays. . . . I have received only partial payment toward rebuilding my house. . . . I have not received any payment for personal losses. Why do I have the feeling that I must beg and grovel for what is rightfully mine? At the age of 79 it is most frightening.

There are three features particular to the San Francisco Bay Area that affected the response to the Loma Prieta earthquake: 1) the multiethnic mixture of the region, 2) the budgetary crisis that mental health programs were facing in 1989, and 3) the extensive media coverage.

Multiethnic Mixture

There are many refugees from Southeast Asia and Central America who have left war-torn countries in which they had experienced multiple traumas. There is a large Asian community from the Philippines, China, and Japan, as well as a large Hispanic population from Mexico. The mental health worker must be sensitive to the cultural and linguistic needs of these populations.

Budgetary Crisis

Throughout the decade, mental health funding had been a low priority for the state. At the time of the earthquake, most community mental health centers (CMHCs) were both understaffed and underfunded. (The previous year, the Public Citizen's Health Research Group ranked California 25th nationally for its quality of public care for those who are seriously mentally ill.) Few of the 10 affected counties had an overall disaster plan. No structure existed to integrate public and private cooperation.

Extensive Media Coverage

Broadcast teams and journalists were already in the Bay Area to cover the World Series. The media made a quick transition from sportscasting to documentary, providing endless coverage of the crushed I-880 freeway, the damaged Bay Bridge, the San Francisco Marina fires, the Santa Cruz mall, and the faces of victims and those who were homeless. Repeated reliving of the disaster via the media intensified reactions, and more vulnerable populations, especially children, were traumatized by what they saw and heard. The news was so sensationalized that many people residing outside of the Bay Area believed that the region had been destroyed, severely affecting the area's economy and tourism in the ensuing months. Even local residents were uncertain of the damage. The *San Francisco Chronicle*, in its headline of October 18, 1989, announced "Hundreds Dead in Huge Quake." The copy described a "terrifying earthquake" that had "ripped through Northern California yesterday afternoon killing more than 200, injuring hundreds, setting buildings ablaze, and destroying sections of the Bay Bridge."

In this chapter, we examine the mental health response to the earthquake by both the public and private sectors. The CMHCs of San Francisco and Santa Cruz counties provide the model of the public sector response. The local psychiatric branch of the American Psychiatric Association (APA) demonstrates the private sector volunteer effort.

Private Sector Response

The Northern California Psychiatric Society

The local APA district branch, the Northern California Psychiatric Society (NCPS), is a volunteer organization of more than 1,300 psychiatrists. The NCPS's geographic boundaries extend southward from the Oregon border to San Luis Obispo. The district branch had neither a disaster plan nor available contingency funding. Nevertheless, immediate work by the salaried executive director and staff, together with the public relations consultant, the chairs of the Public Information and Child and Adolescent Committees, and the NCPS president, led to the development of an earthquake response.

The district branch designed a three-pronged effort that included 1) a media educational component, 2) a telephone hot line, and 3) an outreach program to schools and businesses. Media contacts were established immediately to provide public information and the telephone number of the hot line. Within 48 hours of the earthquake a crisis counseling hot line was in operation at the NCPS headquarters in San Francisco. Within 72 hours the school outreach program began.

The president of the district branch sent a letter to all members informing them of the program and requesting volunteers for the hot line, the "speaker's bureau," outreach programs, and office-based psychotherapy. Voluntary donations to support the program were solicited. Approximately 250 members responded. A list was compiled of "'89 Earthquake Recovery Program Volunteers" for each of the affected counties. An orientation package was prepared for hot line and school consultant volunteers.

Special stationery was designed to give the '89 Earthquake Recovery Program a unique identity and gain access to newsrooms. This stationery identified NCPS as an APA component.

Three temporary staff members were hired to supplement the three full-time staff members and one part-time staff member. Staff were carefully observed for stress reactions during the postquake period. NCPS headquarters adapted to the program needs by modifying the existing computer software. Two new phone lines were installed for the hot line. The conference room was made available for earthquake activities, and two new work stations for computers were added. NCPS spent approximately $8,000 for the programs, allocated to temporary help, the public relations consultant, printing and postage, and additional phone lines. The expenses were defrayed in part by members' donations, a local school donation, and funding from the state society (California Psychiatric Association/Area 6, of which NCPS is one of the five district branches).

The Media

Communication with the media played an integral role in the successful operation of the NCPS's programs. Television, radio, and newspapers disseminated the hot line telephone number. Members were available to the public to answer questions about expected and abnormal responses to the earthquake. Public service announcements and press releases were circulated. Once the activities of the NCPS were announced, schools, businesses, additional media sources, and agencies called to request consultations.

The positive relationship with the media had been established 4 years earlier. The Public Information Committee, appreciating the need for a long-term interaction with the media, began publishing "Media Briefs"—psychiatric updates appearing six times per year, sent to more than 600 media locations in the San Francisco Bay Area. Articles featured such topics as new research, the "holiday blues," and the homeless. Each Media Brief contained three to four articles written by NCPS members, who indicated their availability to talk about the subjects presented. The second key ingredient of the media effort, a speaker's bureau, was composed of psychiatrists prepared to speak with the media and other community groups, often on very limited notice.

The earthquake was an enormous media event, and NCPS received calls from as far away as India and Australia. Members participated in newspaper, television, and radio interviews on both local and national programs. The chairs of the Child and Adolescent Committee were asked to help design public service announcements, and the chair of the Public Information Committee took part in a coast-to-coast hookup on the "MacNeil-Lehrer News Hour" with his counterpart involved in Hurricane Hugo.

There is a negative side to media coverage, particularly its traumatizing effect on more vulnerable populations. There is little one can do to prevent reporters and journalists from sensationalizing events. Our best course is to accept media coverage for what it is, and work as effectively as possible within its boundaries.

Hot Line

The NCPS hot line was in operation for a 15-day period from October 19 through November 2, 1989. During that period, 49 volunteer psychiatrists and mental health workers in 2- to 4-hour shifts logged in more than 145 hours, working weekdays 9 A.M. to 9 P.M. and weekends 9 A.M. to 6 P.M. The earthquake occurred on Tuesday evening and by Thursday the first seven calls were received after the Public Information Committee and public relations team released the hot line phone number to the radio, television, and press. By the end of that first weekend, 81 calls had been received, and another 193 followed in the first Monday-to-Friday period. The number of calls dropped to 76 in the second week, and the hot line was then discontinued.

The great majority of callers were women (81%), often calling about their children (19%) or themselves (71%). Two-thirds of the callers expressed feelings of anxiety and/or fearfulness; one-quarter described sleeping problems; and smaller numbers worried about gastrointestinal symptoms, depression, or their work. Volunteers referred more than half the callers to support groups or therapists and mailed pamphlets from APA (on posttraumatic stress disorder; American Psychiatric Association 1988) and NCPS. The following vignette from one of the volunteer psychiatrists (Plotinsky 1989, p. 3) is representative:

> The most memorable call I received during the two sessions of the hot line was on Sunday, October 29, almost 2 weeks after the earthquake itself. It came from a young woman—all my callers were women—and she presented in the manner quite similar to the presentation of nearly every other caller I spoke with. Her speech was pressured and she frequently had to interrupt herself to take a deep breath or shed a

few tears. Her experiences were most dystonic and she stated clearly that she was behaving differently than she had ever behaved before, and felt different than at any time she could remember.

She told me that she and her husband had recently bought their first house in anticipation of the birth of their first child. One month prior to the earthquake she suddenly had a miscarriage. Although she and her husband were very disappointed, they did manage to rally and had begun to put their lives together again and to anticipate another pregnancy. The earthquake struck, devastating the new home. Friends who had sustained little damage were exceedingly generous and offered the caller and her husband a place to stay while her home was being repaired. But this is when another problem surfaced: the caller was a social worker, and she described herself to me as one who helped others who were in need, not one who accepts help from others.

Most of my conversation with her was aimed at giving her the opportunity to ventilate. I also reassured her that her feelings, though strange to her, were by no means unusual after the events of the past few weeks. I have frequently thought about this conversation with the listener, and wondered how many of us were manning hot lines as a way of dealing with our own strong feelings about the earthquake of '89.

The hot line was a makeshift operation to respond to a crisis. Data collection was minimized in favor of reassurance, support, and education. The lack of statistics makes it difficult to evaluate the effectiveness of the overall operation. Much of the literature on disasters covers the period several weeks to months after the event, and the acute operation of the hot line would have provided much valuable disaster data. Volunteers clearly felt that the callers found the hot line helpful. We were concerned, however, about the ability of the hot line to reach some of the more vulnerable victims, such as inner-city residents without their own telephones and Southeast Asian and Central American refugees with previous traumatic experience and limited English fluency for telephone use. In this sense the hot line must be viewed as one of many emergency measures. Certain individuals preferred the anonymity and easy access of the telephone, and perhaps there were in this group many vulnerable individuals who would not go to a clinic or counseling center.

To prepare for the possible need to establish another hot line in the future, the NCPS is currently developing a standardized hot line data collection sheet. We are particularly interested in finding more bilingual mental health workers. We are also considering ways to use the NCPS hot line specifically for especially vulnerable groups, such as people who have a history of mental disorder or who are receiving psychiatric medications, people with a history of trauma, veterans, elderly people, refugees, and parents whose children are at risk.

Responses to Children and Adolescents

The co-chairs of the NCPS Committee on Children and Adolescents joined with the California Regional Organization of Child and Adolescent Psychiatrists to address the needs of youth. In addition to the hot line and media consultation described earlier in this chapter, efforts were directed to the development of educational materials and consultation to schools. More information may be found elsewhere (Newman 1976; Pynoos and Eth 1984; Terr 1981). In addition, readers are referred to Baisen and Quarantelli's (1981) social service delivery model and the conceptualizations by Auerbach and Spirito (1986) and Pynoos and Nader (1990) on the phases of mental health disaster response intervention.

The NCPS committee co-chairs developed four pamphlets for children, teachers, and mental health professionals. An initial *Facts for Parents: Helping Your Child With the Earthquake* was written by one of us (Ponton 1989a) in collaboration with Dr. Lenore Terr and was modeled after the American Academy of Child and Adolescent Psychiatry *Facts for Families* series handout to facilitate parents' understanding of their children's reactions and coping strategies. The demand for this pamphlet was so great that more than 10,000 copies were printed. It was followed 1 week later by *Helping Your Children After the Earthquake . . . A Long Term Proposition* (Ponton 1989b). A third pamphlet, which was developed for teachers (Northern California Psychiatric Society 1989), offered practical advice and methods to help schoolchildren express their feelings via storytelling, role playing, art and class projects, and disaster preparedness. A final pamphlet was written for mental health professionals, assisting them in educating families, consulting to schools, staffing the hot line, and collaborating with other workers.

More than 15,000 copies of these four pamphlets were disseminated in the community. The timing was serendipitous: the Huntsville tornado struck the following month, and these handouts were readily available for workers in Alabama. The American Academy of Child and Adolescent Psychiatry (1990) has since developed a *Facts for Families* brochure on coping with disasters.

The direct "hands on" work of the Academy of Child and Adolescent Psychiatry is exemplified in the consultation done by six members to a San Francisco school of 400 students, grades kindergarten through eight.

The school principal contacted NCPS headquarters 2 weeks after the earthquake, requesting psychiatric consultation to parents and students. This school had not been physically damaged by the earthquake, but the children had all been exposed to the extensive media coverage, and many had visited the severely affected Marina district. Almost all families had experienced initial power failures, and some had been displaced due to home damage. Many families had been involved in the volunteer rescue effort.

A program was offered that featured a one-day school consultation. In the first hours of the consultation, attended by parents and mental health workers, an educational and informational talk was given followed by questions from parents. The main concerns focused on separation anxiety, sleep disturbances, media impact, and general stress response of the children.

The consultants met with the younger children in small groups of 25 and with the third to eighth graders in groups of less than 50 in a less than 1-hour session. Teaching techniques used involved circle talk, drawing, team games, and discussion. The younger children demonstrated a sense of urgency and anxiety to report their experiences. Their drawings were of fire engines, damaged buildings, and collapsed highways. The smaller group allowed the consultants to identify more symptomatic children.

Children 8 and 9 years old demonstrated magical thinking in their avoidance of discussing the earthquake for fear that it might recur. The mastery of helplessness was a predominant theme. Children 11 and 12 years old expressed anger at Marina "rubberneckers," with some expressing survivor guilt. The older students in grades seven and eight were more verbal and able to talk about their anxieties.

The reaction of the teachers was mixed, from enthusiasm to anger or denial of any need for outsiders. Some felt the intervention was too late, as it occurred 1 month after the earthquake. Their response seemed to reflect their own emotional states and recent administrative changes in the school.

Public Sector Response

San Francisco Community Mental Health Services

The San Francisco Community Mental Health Department—Division of Mental Health, Substance Abuse and Forensic Services (DMSF) began immediately after the earthquake to respond to the trauma. DMSF received grants from the Federal Emergency Management Administration (FEMA) and the National Institute of Mental Health, as well as the state of California Department of Mental Health, in 6-month and subsequent 9-month installments.

Damage to the city and county was random, with maximal damage, predictably, at the Marina district, an area built on landfill after the 1936 World's Fair. Here, 60 buildings were destroyed, and fires burned out of control. The downtown inner city lost nearly 1,000 units that housed mainly poor and immigrant families. The southwest corner of the city, near Lake Merced, lost many senior housing units. Chinatown, in the northern corner, sustained significant structural damage. In all, 13 people died, more than 1,000 were injured, and 421 were hospitalized. Electric power was shut down in many areas of the city. Natural gas supply was stopped.

More than 30,000 San Franciscans received services from the San Francisco public health sector in the first 9 months, and more than 43,000 received services in the 15 months after the earthquake. The role of the DMSF was to provide mental health services in the Red Cross shelters and to deliver outreach and crisis intervention to the community. In the first weeks, six shelters opened and closed. A shelter for senior citizens was established at a local high school immediately after the earthquake, staffed by DMSF geriatric team members and other community mental health workers from local catchment areas. That shelter closed within days. The Moscone Convention Center was opened as a primary shelter serving the inner city and the downtown area and closed within a week. A third shelter also opened immediately after the earthquake, located in the Marina Middle School. Three additional shelters opened: one aboard the USS *Pelieu,* a second at the Army's San Francisco Presidio base, and a third at a former Pierce-Arrow showroom.

The frequent moves were very unsettling to the shelter residents. One example of the general anxiety involved the issuance of yellow hospital wristbands to people sent to the newly opened Presidio shelter from the closing Moscone Center. Rumors went back and forth whether the wristband wearers were to be sheltered or excluded. The Moscone shelter was nearing a panic state until DMSF workers provided yellow wristbands to anyone who wanted one and started wearing them as well.

The general shelter environment was highly stressful. Many of the residents were tearful, anxious, confused, and disorganized, with many somatic complaints. The population was often a heterogeneous mix, although attempts were made to allocate space to families with children, seniors, and those with disabilities. Mental health workers did their best to ease the general dysphoria and to keep the shelters as calm as possible by individual and group counseling and crisis intervention. The shelters established mental health areas where some medications were dispensed, and privacy for individual meetings was available.

> Barbara, a 30-year-old Caucasian female, was 5 months pregnant. She worried about her husband, who had been in the shelter and who had left to see if he could get back into the condemned hotel. Anxious and vulnerable in the shelter environment, she told how the walls came falling in on her. Eventually, she moved to the area for women and children and was able to talk freely there about her experiences.

CMHC personnel worked well with the Red Cross teams. Mental health workers were trusted, and their help was valued. The DMSF team was supplemented by nonprofit contract agency mental health staff, volunteer private mental health workers, mutual aid teams from nearby Napa State Hospital, and mental health workers from less affected areas in California.

A second major area of effort was directed at community outreach and crisis intervention. Vulnerable populations were targeted as a priority. These populations included current clients of the mental health system, elderly people, children, mentally ill people, homeless people, Vietnam veterans, and refugees from Southeast Asia and Central America. The outreach effort was door-to-door, directed at those neighborhoods that had sustained significant damage. Outreach materials were printed in English, Spanish, Chinese, Vietnamese, Russian, and other languages.

> Shortly after the earthquake, Bill, a 39-year-old black Vietnam veteran, requested help from a project agency for housing. His home had been

considerably damaged. During a discussion with the outreach worker, Bill disclosed that his posttraumatic stress disorder symptoms—nightmares from the war—were recurring and that his alcohol consumption had increased. The agency was able to arrange housing for him for 30 days, helped him to enter a residential alcohol treatment program, and subsequently got him into a special program for Vietnam veterans with posttraumatic stress disorder.

DMSF staff also provided outreach to schools, working closely with teachers and principals to identify children at risk. Children spoke with the outreach team of their fears of separation from their parents as well as their fearfulness of loud noises. Parents were encouraged to talk with their children about the earthquake, rather than avoiding a subject they believed to be too traumatic. Clearly, the home visits and outreach were beneficial. Had mental health workers followed more traditional models of waiting for patients to come to their offices, many traumatized individuals would not have received services.

Community Mental Health Efforts in Santa Cruz County

Santa Cruz County, 80 miles south of San Francisco, with a population of 230,000, was severely damaged by the October 17th earthquake. The epicenter was in the county's Nisene Marks State Park at Loma Prieta Mountain. Four people died and 9,000 were dislodged from their homes. In October and November of 1989, 4,000 new unemployment claims, a 400% increase, were filed. Much structural damage was sustained to many old unreinforced masonry buildings, reaffirming the adage, "Earthquakes don't kill people, buildings do."

In the city of Santa Cruz, three large welfare hotels were destroyed, leaving their elderly residents homeless. The picturesque downtown Pacific Garden Mall was gutted, with 32 buildings demolished. The downtown area lost 206 of its 600 businesses; 400 jobs were lost as well. Earthquake damage to the city is conservatively estimated at $115 million.

Nearby Watsonville was especially hard hit. This community of 30,000 includes many Latino migrant farm workers, and there is much poverty and unemployment, as well as housing shortages—all of which worsened after the earthquake. Fourteen hundred persons were left homeless, although for some the Red Cross shelters were an upgrade from previous living conditions. Many distrusted the authorities and refused intervention, erecting a tent city at Callahan Park. Social problems such as drug and alcohol abuse and family violence increased after the earthquake. The school district reported an increased number of dropouts in Latino and immigrant families. A 300% increase in sexual assaults against women was reported by Santa Cruz Vice Mayor Jane Yokoyama at the national earthquake conference 1 year later (Yokoyama 1989).

Estimates of demolition in Watsonville alone exceeded $3 million, including 22 commercial buildings in the downtown area and 52 homes. As of this writing, the unincorporated areas of the county have already seen the demolition of 400 properties, with 100 pending and another 300 in review. A $500 million bridge is to be demolished and replaced.

The city of Santa Cruz was one of the better prepared areas for the emergency and mental health effort. The city fire chief had conducted regular drills. The city had a disaster planning section, and heads of city government departments were given freedom of operation. The CMHC had had a disaster team in readiness since the flood and mud slides of 1983. The CMHC was quickly granted $1.2 million by FEMA, and Project COPE (Counseling Ordinary People in Emergencies) was reborn. Project COPE was a coordinated effort of CMHC and private mental health workers to assist people recovering from trauma. Project COPE included community recovery groups, individual family counseling and/or consultations, group presentations, and school outreach consultation. The city of Santa Cruz had a school intervention model, and Watsonville likewise had a school plan.

The CMHC coordinated efforts of the health department, the county emergency operation center, the state Department of Mental Health, and private practitioners. Additional staff members were needed to supplement the understaffed CMHC programs as well as to deal with the bilingual population and the extensive emotional stress from the damage. Private-sector psychiatrists, psychologists, social workers, and counselors were recruited for the 12 shelters or to provide office-based treatment. In the first 6 weeks, 10–30 clinicians from nonaffected areas came daily to the county. Trauma consultants from the Veterans Hospital volunteered and established a clinic that was open for 1 year. Spanish-speaking therapists were contacted to work specifically with the Watsonville population and to provide bilingual printed material.

Victims were seen individually, in family units, and in groups at drop-in centers, shelters, offices, or in their homes. Countywide debriefing was provided for city rescue personnel and mental health workers. Project COPE issued public service announcements about expected traumatic responses and met with the media to inform and educate the public. A telephone hot line was installed by the third day after the earthquake.

As the aftershocks continued, so too did the stress responses. In the first month after the earthquake, 24 aftershocks measuring over 4.0 on the Richter scale were recorded. Predictions by "experts" further alarmed residents. CMHC staff described that bipolar patients were increasingly manic but helpful in the community; depressive patients were less depressed; and schizophrenic patients were often more delusional, at times seeing the event as a sign from God. Borderline character disorder patients tended to be more dysfunctional, with increased substance abuse. Victims of previous traumata were at especially high risk.

Project COPE also reached the schools. Fortunately, the earthquake occurred after school hours, when students were already safely at home. Team members wrote to school district supervisors explaining their services. Follow-up calls were made in a week or two, requesting a contact person. Face-to-face meetings were then held with that contact person, and written materials were provided to be used by staff, students, and parents. Team members then met with individual teachers to discuss needs and problems of the particular school, such as violence or drug abuse, and to clarify treatment goals. Finally, teams went into the schools, fully informed about demographics of the population, after the path had been cleared and initial resistance overcome. Project COPE members always remembered to regard themselves as guests in the schools and treated their hosts with the utmost respect.

Epilogue

The earthquake was followed by many proposals and promises. Architectural grants, soil studies, and budgetary allotments for additional fire trucks, ambulances, and backup generators were the order of the day. The legislature introduced more than 400 earthquake safety bills. Gov-

ernor Deukmejian signed into law SB 2902, mandating statewide earthquake insurance protection. The economy and tourism began to improve, although many local residents missed the newly available
downtown parking, affordable luxury hotels, and previously unobtain-
able restaurant reservations. By the summer after the Loma Prieta
earthquake, the Bay Area had returned to its prequake complacency. A
survey of chief executive officers, senior executives, and commercial
property owners conducted in July 1990 rated "earthquake risk" least
important of 10 possible factors affecting selection of a site for business
expansion or relocation. In fact, "almost half (48%) of the business
executives surveyed, and nearly three-quarters (72.5%) of the commercial property professionals said the overall impact of the earthquake on
their firms was negligible" (Bay Area Council 1990, p. 1).

Newspaper polls conducted on the first anniversary of the earthquake were similarly buoyant. The *San Francisco Chronicle* ("*Chronicle* Earthquake Poll" 1990) found that only 16% of its readers "worry
very much" about another major earthquake, compared to twice that
figure at the time of the event. The *Marin Independent Journal* (October 17, 1990, p. 6) surveyed 500 telephone respondents in its story
"Quake No Big Deal," commenting "nearly half, one year later, said the
earthquake had little or no effect on their lives." Although 80% believed another earthquake was likely, 78% said they would remain and
rebuild.

Overall, the Bay Area responded well to the earthquake, and its
minimal damage is a testament to the general good structural design.
Predictably, unreinforced masonry buildings, bridges, and soft soil (the
site of the Marina fires and freeway deaths) were the main problem
areas. Nevertheless, many people are still homeless and psychologically traumatized. Many small businesses and housing units have been
lost. Many individuals continue to wade through the bureaucratic process of receiving compensation for their lost homes.

The Loma Prieta earthquake was a warning to heed. The California
Division of Mines and Geology commented that had the epicenter
occurred closer to an urban area, one could have expected deaths to
reach 4,500 and injuries to surpass 100,000 (Ward and Page 1989). In
fact, seismologists now predict, with odds of 2:1, that the region will
experience another major quake in the next 30 years.

The earthquake taught the mental health community that it needs
to be prepared and have plans ready. The earthquake is behind us, but

not its lessons. As the Persian Gulf War began in January 1991, the Bay Area reexperienced the anxiety of those postquake days—but this time the community was alerted, with plans to use the tools from the 1989 San Francisco Bay Area earthquake.

References

American Academy of Child and Adolescent Psychiatry: Facts for Families: Coping With Disasters. Washington, DC, American Academy of Child and Adolescent Psychiatry, 1990

American Psychiatric Association: Let's Talk Facts About Post-traumatic Stress Disorder. Washington, DC, American Psychiatric Association, 1988

Auerbach AL, Spirito A: Crisis intervention with children exposed to natural disasters, in Crisis Intervention With Children and Families. Edited by Auerbach SM, Stolberg AL. New York, McGraw-Hill, 1986

Baisen D, Quarantelli E: The delivery of mental health services in community disaster: an outline of research finding. Journal of Community Psychology 9:195–203, 1981

Bay Area Council: Earthquake Survey. San Francisco, CA, Bain & Co, July 1990, p 1

Chronicle earthquake poll. San Francisco Chronicle, October 17, 1990, p A1

Hundreds dead in huge quake. San Francisco Chronicle, October 18, 1989, p 1

Lindh A: Loma Prieta earthquake. Paper presented at Putting the Pieces Together: A National Conference About the Loma Prieta Earthquake: One Year Later, San Francisco, CA, October 16, 1990

Newman CJ: Children of disaster: clinical observations at Buffalo Creek. Am J Psychiatry 133:306–312, 1976

Northern California Psychiatric Society: Facts for Teachers: Helping Children After the Earthquake. San Francisco, CA, Northern California Psychiatric Society, 1989

Plakker G, Galloway JP (eds): Lessons learned from the Loma Prieta, California, earthquake of October 17, 1989 (U.S. Geological Survey Circular 1045). Washington, DC, U.S. Government Printing Office, 1989, p 1

Plotinsky I: Days on the quake hot line. Northern California Psychiatric Physician, December 1989, p 3

Ponton L: Facts for Parents: Helping Your Child With the Earthquake, Part I. San Francisco, CA, Northern California Psychiatric Society, 1989a

Ponton L: Facts for Parents: Helping Your Child After the Earthquake . . . A Long-Term Proposition, Part II. San Francisco, CA, Northern California Psychiatric Society, 1989b

Pynoos RS, Eth S: The child as witness to homicide. Journal of Social Issues 40:87–108, 1984

Pynoos RS, Nader K: Mental health disturbances in children exposed to disaster: prevention intervention strategies, in Preventing Mental Health Disturbances in Childhood. Edited by Goldston SE, Yager J, Heinicke CM, et al. Washington, DC, American Psychiatric Press, 1990, pp 211–234

Quake no big deal. Marin Independent Journal, October 17, 1990

Reaction of the public. San Francisco Examiner, October 19, 1989, p A6

Terr L: Psychic trauma in children: observations following the Chowchilla school bus kidnapping. Am J Psychiatry 138:14–19, 1981

Ward P, Page R: The Loma Prieta earthquake of October 17, 1989 (U.S. Geological Survey Pamphlet 11-1989). Washington, DC, U.S. Geological Survey, 1989, p 7

Williamson M: Letter to the editor. San Jose Mercury News, October 14, 1990, p 1A

Yokoyama J: Elected officials' perspectives on Loma Prieta. Paper presented at Putting the Pieces Together: A National Conference about the Loma Prieta Earthquake: One Year Later, San Francisco, CA, October 16, 1989

Chapter 9

The Armenian Earthquake

Haikaz M. Grigorian, M.D., F.A.P.A.

*O*n December 7, 1988, at 11:41 A.M. Soviet Armenian time, an earthquake of 6.9 magnitude on the Richter scale occurred in northern Armenia. When the earthquake struck, children were in school, and adults were at their places of employment.

To understand the impact of the earthquake, it is important to understand the history of the area. Armenia is a mountainous land as large as Maryland and is bordered by Turkey and Iran. Its population is 3.5 million. The earthquake struck the northern part of Armenia, including the cities Leninakan, Stepanavan, Kirovakan, and Spitak. Armenia was one of the 15 republics of the former Soviet Union. Before 1920, it was an independent republic but was subsequently annexed by the Soviet Union. From 1920 to 1991, the Armenians of Karabagh, comprising 85% of the population, were annexed to the former Soviet Republic of Azerbaijan. Under the Soviet Azerbaijan rule, Armenians were not able to promulgate their language and culture or worship in Armenian churches. In February 1988 the Karabagh Armenians, inspired by the spirit of glasnost, voted to request of the Supreme Soviet that they be detached from Azerbaijan and annexed to Soviet Armenia. The population of Armenia was tense with anticipation, hopes, and dreams, as well as frustration, waiting for the Supreme Soviet to make that decision. In response to the annexation movement, atrocities had been committed against Armenians in the Azerbaijan cities of Baku and Sumgait. Many Armenians had escaped to Armenia, eventually to become earthquake victims.

Armenia became an independent republic after the dissolution of the Soviet Union. On March 2, 1992, the Republic of Armenia became a member of the United Nations. Karabagh Armenians continue their struggle with Azerbaijan, and there has been no annexation with Armenia.

At the time the earthquake struck, half a world away, Mikhail Gorbachev, the Soviet premier, was making a speech at the United Nations in New York City. A group of 5,000 Armenian Americans of the New York metropolitan area had gathered on the grounds of St. Vartan Cathedral in New York City to demonstrate solidarity through prayers with the Armenians of the world, in hopes that President Gorbachev would notice this public outpouring of support for their homeland. When the announcement of the earthquake was made at the demonstration, the group was stunned and fell silent. No one knew the magnitude of the disaster, but that evening when President Gorbachev decided to interrupt his visit and return to the Soviet Union, it was clear that this was not an ordinary earthquake but a major disaster.

For the first time in the 70-year history of the Soviet Union, the foreign news media was given free access to the disaster area, in contrast to the secrecy that shrouded the Chernobyl nuclear disaster. This resulted in an outpouring of assistance to Armenia, including 300 planeloads of medical and rescue supplies from 90 different countries within the first 48 hours. The Armenian American community began to mobilize itself to gather funds and emergency supplies. The initial concern was to save lives by rescuing people from beneath the rubble. The next concern was to house the 500,000 people who were left homeless in the middle of the winter. Concern about the mental health of those exposed to the disaster followed later.

The Land and Culture Organization is an international organization that addresses itself to preservation of Armenian culture and antiquities. In January 1989, as a board member of the Land and Culture Organization, I and two other board members were asked to go to Armenia to explore the possibility of our volunteers participating in the reconstruction effort.

I arrived in Yerevan, the capital of Armenia, on January 28, 1989, and the following day was given a tour of the devastated area. The magnitude of the destruction reminded me of the pictures of Hiroshima and Nagasaki. The Minister of Health of Soviet Armenia, Dr. Emil Gabrielian, gave us the statistics on the human casualties as well as property damages. The estimated population of the earthquake disaster area was 750,000. The death toll was over 25,000, with an additional 327 amputations, 200 spinal cord injuries, and 17,000 other injuries. Destroyed were 84 hospitals, 380 schools and universities, and 84 million square feet of housing. In comparison, the October 1989 San Francisco earthquake, which was of the same magnitude in a population center of 8 million, resulted in 67 deaths and 12,000 homeless. Leninakan, the second largest city in Armenia with a population of 300,000, was half destroyed. Spitak, population 20,000, was completely destroyed. Stepanavan and Kirovakan were partially destroyed, and 58 villages disappeared completely. Because of the destruction of factories and collective industries, 170,000 people were left jobless. The financial damage was estimated at 16 billion rubles. It was estimated that each survivor of the earthquake had lost at least 10 relatives. Since I had been involved in the treatment of survivors of the Armenian genocide of 1915–1923, I anticipated inevitable depression and posttraumatic stress disorder.

My first 2 days were spent visiting the children's hospitals. I was accompanied by three orthopedic surgeons from Project Hope in the United States who selected children to be brought to the United States for specialized surgery and rehabilitation. Drs. Dennis Carroll, Dennis Drummond, and John Remensnyder interviewed children and available relatives. Children with all types of complex orthopedic injuries needed specialized surgery unavailable to them in Armenia. Since assistance was needed to take histories and explain physical examinations, my help as an interpreter was welcome, allowing me to observe the psychological implications of injuries and hospitalization. I was impressed by the compliance and cooperation of the children and their ability to tolerate pain. In time, some of the children displayed eating difficulties, nightmares, and withdrawn behavior.

It is customary in Armenia that a member of the family stays with a hospitalized child, feeding, cleaning, comforting, and sleeping next to the child. Project Hope planned to bring relatives with the children to the United States, which was a salutary and sensitive response to the situation. It was obvious that these children were precious to the staff. Since the genocide of 1915–1923, children have a special place in Armenian families, and most of them were named after relatives who had perished. The Soviet government's decision to take some of the injured children outside Armenia resulted in public protest that this was a deliberate attempt to displace the children and assimilate them into other nationalities. The staff, including pediatricians, surgeons, and nurses, were somber and occasionally tearful, working nonstop for days, under emotionally tense, technically limited circumstances. Some staff had lost relatives and were grief stricken.

While in Armenia I tried to determine whether any Armenian mental health professionals were aware of the need for mental health services. Clinical psychologists were rare, and typically psychiatrists confined themselves to the biological treatment of patients with major psychiatric disorders, either inpatient or posthospitalization. There were no social workers or psychotherapists, and psychologists were confined to pedagogical institutes (teacher's colleges).

I was able to meet Prof. Emma Alexandryan, who had received her Ph.D. from Moscow University and who taught an elementary school education section of Apovian Pedagogical Institute. I observed her working with children who were brought from earthquake zones to live in Yerevan temporarily. Some of the children were in the acute phase of trauma. By comforting and holding the children, she helped them verbalize and draw what had happened during the earthquake. Invariably in their drawings, the children depicted the destroyed buildings and began to talk slowly and cautiously about their present situation. A brother and sister seen separately talked about their present school and living situations, but were silent about their mother, who had died in the earthquake. It became evident that a large number of children were traumatized and displaced and needed psychological intervention. Entire classrooms with children had vanished in the earthquake, and the surviving children had lost cousins and often parents. These children struggled to master the trauma and resolve survival guilt in the months that followed.

In the meantime, a curfew was established in Yerevan, and Soviet troops and tanks occupied key streets to prevent unrest. Groups of Armenians, primarily men, gathered in public squares to talk about atrocities in Baku and Sumgait. Some were refugees from those areas who speculated about the outcome of the struggle. Other groups formed around places where homeless people could receive clothing and supplies that were being distributed and talked about their present predicament. People spontaneously gathered to commiserate about the two major contemporary calamities of their lives: the Karabagh conflict and the earthquake. It would have been a natural opportunity to start self-help groups by mental health professionals.

The response of the Armenian population to the earthquake can be understood only in the context of the unresolved Karabagh conflict. Gorbachev's visit to Armenia as a sympathetic leader wishing to share his sorrow was completely misinterpreted and misunderstood by the Armenians, who were rude, hostile, and inhospitable. Rumors spread that the earthquake was caused by the Soviet explosion of an atom bomb under the city of Kirovakan to punish Armenians for creating the Karabagh conflict. If the Karabagh conflict had not existed, the country might have been able to proceed more quickly with reconstruction.

A joke illustrates the important tie between the Karabagh conflict and the earthquake. An old man was dug out of the rubble of Leninakan alive. After he recovered, the first question he asked was not about his wife, children, or grandchildren, but whether the Karabagh conflict was resolved. When he was told "No," he threw his arms in the air and said, "Bury me again." This illustrates that people's preoccupation about an unresolved previous conflict drained energy that could have been used to restore their lives.

The two nations that have had the greatest impact on the Armenian psyche during the last century were Turkey and Russia, and they played an important role in the earthquake response. The Turkish people, which includes the Azeris, were regarded as persecutors, starting in the 1890s with a series of mass killings of Armenians by the Turkish people and culminating in the 1915–1923 genocide. The 1915 atrocities left the Armenians stigmatized as "the starving Armenians," and "the poor, helpless, victimized Armenians." On the other hand, the Russian people have been traditionally perceived by some Armenians as benefactors and saviors, starting with the Czars Alexander III and Nicholas II and ending with the Soviet Union's Lenin, Stalin, Khrushchev, Brezhnev, Andropov, and finally Gorbachev. However, because of 70 years of Soviet rule, there was ambivalence and mistrust. In the past, every time an event threatened the existence of Armenia, the Russians and the Turks had an important role to play in the Armenian psyche.

There is a new force that is a part of the Armenian psyche: the Armenian diaspora (i.e., Armenian communities formed outside the homeland as a result of dispersion). After the Karabagh conflict and the earthquake, the Armenian diaspora became mobilized, unified, and willing to participate in the creation of a new Armenia. The caring and support of the diaspora has been a source of hope and inspiration to Armenians. The Psychiatric Outreach Program is an example of an Armenian diaspora organization from the United States serving Armenia.

The Earthquake Relief Fund of Armenia of the Armenian Relief Society and the California Armenian American Medical Association

provided financial assistance for mental health services in Armenia.
Sixty mental health professionals of Armenian ancestry—including
Armenian-speaking psychiatrists, child psychiatrists, psychologists,
psychiatric social workers, and nurse clinicians—have provided services to 10,000 children, adolescents, and adults beginning in February
1989. The team was lead by Dr. Armen Geonjian, a California-based
psychiatrist. Meline Karakashian, Ed.S., a psychologist who recently
completed her third tour of service in Armenia, reported the following
clinical example, illustrating survivor guilt, which has also been observed in the survivors of the Armenian genocide.

> Mariam, a school-age girl, was seen in group therapy in the city of
> Leninakan, 16 months after the earthquake. In the group she casually
> mentioned that she had attempted suicide 2 weeks previously, jumping
> in front of a car. Her parents were notified, and she was evaluated in
> individual sessions. The reason she gave for her despair was the deaths
> of her 2-year-old cousin and 22 of her 30 classmates in the earthquake.
> She herself was miraculously rescued, and her leg was saved from
> amputation.
>
> The parents of her dead classmates repeatedly asked her how was
> it that she survived and their children did not. Did she know where to
> go in the falling building in order to escape? They made comments to
> her mother such as, "How lucky you are that both your children
> survived. Why couldn't Mariam die and my son be alive?" Her aunt
> who had lost a child would comment frequently, "All the beautiful and
> bright children died. The ugly and the dumb survived." Mariam felt
> guilty for living. After learning of this, Mariam's mother talked to the
> grieving parents, who asked for forgiveness and began to treat Mariam
> more kindly.

In 1989, Dr. Louis M. Najarian, a child psychiatrist from New
York, reported that of 179 patients treated, 72% received a diagnosis of
post-traumatic stress disorder, 8% conversion disorder, and 7% depression (personal communication, September 1989). Dr. Najarian returned
to Armenia for 1 year to train local psychiatrists, psychologists, and
psychotherapists to serve the earthquake survivors. It is estimated that
there is a need for 600 school psychologists to diagnose and treat
children and families in Leninakan, Spitak, Stepanavan, Kirovakan,
and adjoining communities. The Psychiatric Outreach Program will
continue to send teams of mental health professionals to provide indi-

vidual and group therapy as well as psychoeducational presentations to teachers and other groups.

I returned to Armenia in October 1989 accompanied by a psychiatric social worker of Armenian descent on behalf of the Psychiatric Outreach Program. Working in a children's hospital in Leninakan, we treated children individually and in groups with their family members. Most of the children were in the hospital for somatic problems. An increasing number of children were hospitalized for abdominal surgery, gastrointestinal complaints, and idiopathic thrombocytopenic purpura. Concomitantly, some children still complained about nightmares, difficulty sleeping alone at nights, lack of concentration, restlessness in school, and crying. Family members and their children had invariably lost loved ones and continued to talk about the earthquake and their losses. The hospital staff also suffered from depression and symptoms of posttraumatic stress disorder. They spoke of the loss of their relatives and described their own symptoms, including memory impairment, anhedonia, difficulty concentrating, and insomnia. Many children were observed to stutter.

> One 9-year-old boy began to stutter after the earthquake. He had no prior psychiatric history but the stuttering had intensified to a degree that interfered with socialization. His mother reported that he played the "earthquake game" with his friends. The children would make houses in a mound of sand and take turns stomping on the houses. All the mothers interrupted the play and forbade it because it reminded them of the earthquake. On examination the child was normal except he had fears of recurrence of the earthquake. His psychiatrist, Dr. Najarian, explained to the mother the benefit of play because it allowed active mastery of a trauma experienced passively. The mother understood the concept and reluctantly allowed the child to play. In time the stuttering resolved.

As of this writing, the Psychiatric Outreach Program maintains outpatient clinics both in Leninakan and Spitak, providing ongoing mental health services.

In February 1989 and May 1989, we evaluated and treated the patients airlifted for treatment to the United States. The first group of six patients came to the Hospital for Joint Diseases at Beth Israel in New York City. The patients had amputations and spinal cord injuries. Six Armenian-speaking psychiatrists and six psychologists/psychotherapists volunteered to provide supportive therapy for the patients; I led the clinical discussion about these cases. Twenty-five Armenian-speaking volunteers provided around-the-clock companionship to the patients and functioned as interpreters. The first 2 weeks were quite stressful for the patients as they underwent repeated surgery. The volunteers were unfamiliar with the hospital environment and experienced anxiety themselves, feeling helpless in the face of so much pain and suffering. The patients were hypervigilant and were afraid of even venipuncture. Some of them screamed at the sight of blood, were easily startled, and had frequent crying spells. The discussion during our March meeting reflected the volunteers' uncertainty about how to respond to their patients. We encouraged the volunteers to allow the patients to talk about their families in order to work through their losses and depression. Armenian clergy also began to visit. Although as part of the Soviet Union for 70 years Armenia was considered to be an atheist country, the patients seemed to enjoy the clergy visits. Next to each patient's bed a picture of the Catholicos (i.e., the highest-ranking clergyman in the Armenian Apostolic Church) of all Armenians was attached to the wall. A 7-year-old boy with scalp and spinal injuries was asked whether he knew whose picture it was. His immediate response was "Lenin."

S.K. was a 28-year-old married woman who had been 6 months pregnant at the time of the earthquake. Her two daughters, 2 and 4 years old, died in her arms during the disaster. She also had an amputation of her left leg below the hip. She was silent and apathetic and refused to eat. We did not know how to relate to the enormity of her tragedy or how to establish a therapeutic relationship with her. Initially the nurse-psychoanalyst and I confined ourselves to the patient's physical needs and comfort.

Gradually and spontaneously S.K. began to talk about the tragedy. She started writing poetry describing her despair and anger at God. The healing of her stump progressed well postsurgery. She became more interested in her environment and developed relationships with the volunteers who brought home-cooked Armenian food. She continued to write poetry, and the content became less gloomy. She was apprehensive as to how the prosthesis would look and feel and whether her husband would find her attractive. She worried about her sexuality and whether she could become pregnant again. Eventually she was fitted with a prosthesis that she was able to wear comfortably. Follow-up information revealed that she stepped out of the plane in Yerevan Airport holding her head high to greet her waiting husband. She subsequently became pregnant again.

In addition to S.K., I met two survivors, both male amputees who also began to write poetry for the first time. Poetry as an art form appears to have therapeutic value in mastering trauma; Armenian literature is replete with postgenocide writings and poetry.

We were concerned about the quality of life for the amputees in Armenia, where there is stigma attached to being handicapped.

Another patient, N.K., a 26-year-old single woman, had a right below-knee amputation with a fracture dislocation of the left ring finger and a left arm crush injury with scar formation at her left forearm. During her first week of hospitalization she seemed to be interested in her treatment and invested in her future. When the time arrived for the fitting of the prosthesis, she flatly refused to even touch it. I was asked to help. She was bitter, angry, and negativistic, telling me politely not to waste my time with her. The appearance of the prosthesis "disgusted" her, and she would not touch it, let alone attach it to her body. She preferred to be sent back home without the prosthesis. I called a meeting of all the patients who were amputees at different hospitals and who were at different stages of their rehabilitation, hoping that with support from the group she might accept the prosthesis. Ten patients were brought to the meeting, which immediately took on the atmosphere of a social gathering. Some patients were in wheelchairs, some were on crutches and walkers, and others had prostheses. They started to talk to each other and to catch up with each other and news from home. At the end of the session when I offered to meet with them again, they suggested that they would prefer to meet with all the other patients and the volunteers socially, preferring not to be singled out as an amputee group. N.K. subsequently accepted the prosthesis and further therapeutic interventions.

Recent follow-up information indicates satisfactory adjustment.

It would be interesting to explore the application of formal group therapy or self-help groups in Armenia. Preliminary attempts have been encouraging. However, freedom of speech has been repressed for 70 years in Armenia. The shadow of the KGB was always felt, making it difficult for patients to be willing to trust each other or for the therapists to speak freely and develop a therapeutic alliance.

The following was reported by Dr. Levon Z. Boyajian, a psychiatrist in New Jersey, where 29 earthquake victims were being treated in different hospitals under the auspices of the Armenian General Benevolent Union, and I served as the chairman of the medical board.

A 29-year-old single man had suffered multiple injuries and was a management problem in the hospital. He refused to continue some of his medications, was uncooperative with the staff, and had difficulty sleeping. His psychiatrist noted that in the initial visit he was "a little bit wary because I had told him I was a psychiatrist." Dr. Boyajian went on to describe the patient: "He displayed an amazing cultural paranoia. He was almost a caricature of someone who had swallowed the Soviet cold war propaganda, hook, line, and sinker. His attitude was essentially that everything was better in the Soviet Union, that we had all forms of deficiencies, and that fundamentally he did not trust any of us in the United States." Later on this patient had difficulties getting along with the housekeeper in the house where he was placed with other compatriots. He was noted to drink excessively. The patient had personality disturbances and suffered posttraumatic stress disorder, but it was helpful that his consultant was an Armenian-speaking psychiatrist.

The above case illustrates the cultural paranoia as well as the role of the psychiatrist as a consultant helping the caretakers. The latter was noticeable in Armenia, where the caretakers needed to understand the behavior of earthquake victims. The mental health professional can make a contribution by helping the caretakers.

In March 1988 I interviewed three other patients from Project Hope who presented with different clinical and behavioral problems.

K.A. was a 14-year-old amputee who refused to leave her room. She would not let her mother out of sight, had stopped eating, had lost weight, and could not tolerate being left alone. On clinical examination she was found to be depressed. A tricyclic antidepressant was prescribed, and she was treated with psychotherapy with an Armenian-speaking therapist.

L.A. was a 15-year-old amputee who was found to have a chronic hearing impairment. She apparently could not understand or cooperate in her rehabilitation. She and her father had difficulty accepting the use of a hearing aid. She was treated supportively and eventually agreed to accept the hearing aid.

D.A. was a 9-year-old boy who would not allow anyone to touch the stump of his left arm below his shoulder. His mother was also apprehensive about the outcome of his rehabilitation. Both were treated supportively, and the patient allowed us to examine the stump. The presence of an Armenian neurosurgeon facilitated the consultation by creating trust and reassurance.

Summary

In this chapter a variety of clinical situations have been illustrated. The cases illustrate the range of the individual responses to the trauma and its behavioral manifestations, as well as the cultural, political, and historic factors impinging on the traumatized people as a group. Clearly, continued clinical services in the traumatized community are essential. Eventually the optimal arrangement would be for care to be delivered by trained indigenous mental health professionals, with consultations provided as needed. It will also be important to collect data to provide a better understanding of the impact of this disaster on the present and future generations in Armenia.

Selected Readings

Davidson S: Transgenerational transmission in the families of holocaust survivors. International Journal of Family Psychiatry 1(1):95–112, 1980

Engholm C: The Armenian Earthquake. San Diego, CA, Lucent Books, 1989

Epstein RS: Post-traumatic stress disorder: a review of diagnostic and treatment issues. Psychiatric Annals 19(10):556–563, 1989

Hovannisian RG (ed): The Armenian Genocide in Perspective. New Brunswick, NJ, Transactions, 1986

Neiderland W: The survivor syndrome: further observations and dimensions. J Am Psychoanal Assoc 29(2):413–425, 1981

Van der Kolk BA: Psychological Trauma. Washington, DC, American Psychiatric Press, 1987

Chapter 10

Forming the Libidinal Cocoon:
The Dallas Airplane Crashes,
the Guadalupe River Drownings,
and Hurricane Hugo in the Virgin Islands

James Black, M.D.

Disasters come in many forms, each leaving a unique signature on a community. This chapter recounts experiences at three very different sorts of disasters: two jet crashes at the Dallas–Fort Worth Airport, a mass drowning of children on a school bus in the Guadalupe River, and the aftereffects of Hurricane Hugo in the Virgin Islands.

The Crash of Delta 191
in Dallas

August is a hot month in Texas, and many people try to leave the state for vacations before school starts in September. Thus, on August 2, 1985, when temperatures climbed to over 100°F, a few rain clouds were welcomed by most residents. Shortly after 6 P.M. on that day, however, the crash of Delta Flight 191 set in motion events that brought back memories of the presidential assassination 24 years before. A huge L1011 jet had become the victim of a microburst cloud and crashed into a giant water tower at the north end of the east runway of Dallas–Fort Worth (DFW) Airport. The crash resulted in 137 immediate deaths and fewer than 30 survivors, most of whom were injured. In the weeks that followed, several of the survivors died of burns and internal trauma. The identification of the body parts of crash victims was expected to take up to a week.

Delta Airlines arranged to fly family members of the victims from all over the country to Dallas and to house these people in a single hotel used exclusively for survivors during that time. The hotel chosen for this was the DFW Hilton, located about 2 miles from the DFW Airport in an isolated area. Designed as a halfway meeting place for firms with offices on either coast, it contained a large number of meeting rooms and had a jogging track and tennis courts outside. No shops or adjacent businesses were near. This made the hotel an ideal psychological retreat, protected from the outside world. If the hotel had been in downtown Dallas, the shops and theaters would have been distracting to the survivors and mourners. If the hotel had been near the Parkland Trauma Center Hospital and the coroner's lab, the pressure to view the body parts of victims of the crash would again have detracted from the grief process.

Working through Parkland Hospital, I volunteered to move into the DFW Hilton for that week to live and work with the surviving families. As a psychiatrist, I orchestrated a sophisticated treatment team to address the psychiatric, medical, and religious needs of the survivors. Working in the hotel with the Red Cross Disaster Cadre (a team of experienced nurses), we established a 24-hour-a-day nursing station complete with medications and a crash cart. A treatment team, consisting of several Red Cross nurses and me, made rounds in the hotel as if it were a hospital. Volunteer clergy from various synagogues and churches conducted services in their faiths and were available for religious consultation as part of the mental health team. Delta Airlines marketing representatives were assigned to each family as facilitators for needs such as replacement of luggage, clothing, and special personal items.

The staff and support system of the entire hotel focused on ministering to the physical and emotional needs of the families. Our goal was to create a protective environment, much as a loving parent provides a small child with shelter, food, clothing, and spiritual and emotional support. The massive trauma fostered a deep regression in most individuals and families, which allowed the mental health team to attend to fundamental emotional issues, often bypassing the usual defenses seen in nontraumatized adults. The term *libidinal cocoon* seemed to conceptualize the effort to provide an isolated, protective environment. The goal was to minister to the anguish of bereavement by allowing a therapeutic regression (Black 1987).

Regression refers to the return to an earlier form of adaptation. This is not to say that an adult under stress acts like a child, although some surely do; rather, some of the defenses used are more typical of early developmental phases. These defenses are mechanisms that serve to protect the person against dangers arising from his or her impulses or feelings. For example, some Delta 191 survivors and families displayed a regression from abstract thinking to attachment to a concrete form or tangible item. One family who lost their mother wanted to have one of their mother's teeth placed in a gold pendant to hang around each family member's neck as a talisman to "keep mother with us at all times." Another family wanted a portable tape player with headphones placed in the intensive care unit so an unconscious family member "could hear." A survivor with a huge abrasion on his leg eagerly came to have me dress his "wound" with full-strength Tincture of Green Soap with 70% alcohol; when the mixture was rubbed into his leg he felt "something" for the first time since the crash. The DSM-III-R (American Psychiatric Association 1987) description of posttraumatic stress disorder (PTSD) notes numbing of general responsiveness to stimuli, and this almost caustic mixture broke through his detachment.

The regression was helpful in allowing the treatment team to become temporary authority figures to protect the fragile state of the families. For example, I would write "prescriptions" that forbade the families to look at the survivors' remains. Most of the caskets were sealed, as the dismembered, charred remains were devoid of human form and would have been profoundly disturbing to the family members. The coroner and I discussed this point at length. The clergy also responded in an authoritative manner. The Orthodox Jewish faith requires that remains be buried by sundown of the first day. The autopsies took 4–5 days in some cases, and the Orthodox Rabbi was helpful in working with these families.

A number of well-known posttraumatic symptoms were predicted for crash survivors, and efforts of the treatment team were structured to minimize these occurrences. For example, the DSM-III-R description of PTSD notes that psychogenic amnesia, an inability to recall important aspects of the trauma, is a frequent symptom. The treatment team attempted to help survivors overcome the distorting effects of amnesia by use of historical logs describing important events surrounding the disaster. Another goal was to protect survivors from potentially exploitative entrepreneurs who could take advantage of mental confusion to pursue commercial enterprises that might not be in the best interest of the survivors. We attempted also to prepare the individual and the family for emergence back into society. We distributed an American Psychiatric Association brochure on PTSD and arranged for survivors' personal physicians to follow the survivors closely. Family education was a paramount concern for the long travail that would follow.

In the 3 years that followed the crash, "Operation Firebird" drills were executed in which the city of Dallas had mock airplane crash drills with several hundred simulated casualties to give fire fighters, paramedics, and caregivers experience in emergency response. The Texas Society of Psychiatric Physicians developed a disaster plan that included on-call psychiatrists of various hospitals going to the emergency room to await casualties or to the crash site. Several meetings with the American Red Cross Disaster team and the Red Cross Nurse Disaster Cadre refined the role of the health care providers at emergencies.

The American Red Cross volunteered its facilities in 1985 for debriefing of those associated with the airplane crash. Fire fighters, police officers, baggage handlers, and airline personnel used one group of debriefings. The nonaffected but interested civilian population was invited to a separate group of debriefings, and the Delta personnel held a third series at their headquarters. A similar group of meetings was held on the 1-year anniversary of the crash in 1986 with good attendance.

A Second Airplane Disaster

On August 31, 1988, at 9:30 A.M., a Delta 727 crashed on takeoff at 50 feet in the air with 108 people aboard. Thirteen people, including two flight attendants, died. For the more than 90 survivors and the families, the DFW Hilton Hotel again was used for its proximity to the airport and its relative isolation. This time many survivors were briefly examined at emergency rooms and sent to the DFW Hilton to receive psychiatric counseling while their casts dried and their burns were being treated.

The two airplane crashes were similar in that the same airport and airline, and some of the same caregivers, were involved. The 1985 crash involved working mainly with the families of the survivors during the identification process; the 1988 crash response involved brief crisis intervention for crash survivors. PTSD was common, and during the following months many survivors returned to the crash site and partic-ipated in desensitization behavioral modification therapy in which they boarded an airplane similar to the one that crashed.

Many survivors of the 1988 crash were ambulatory and in various stages of emotional shock. One curious event was that a group of survivors who wanted to be interviewed on the mobile Minicam televi-sion went into a fugue-like state while telling their stories and began reexperiencing the crash. We gently interrupted the interview.

Paranoid people in an airplane crash often felt a sense of relief as their suspicions were verified. One such individual insisted on keeping a recorder on at all times, making people nervous. I responded to this by introducing myself and each member of the treatment team to him, and we worked with him as a group, never alone.

In the subsequent months, I took several survivors aboard a 727 jet identical to the one that crashed. Although the colors, seating, and interior layout were identical to the plane that crashed, not one survivor thought it was a similar plane. Walking around outside, survivors commented that there were too many or too few jet engines, or that the front end of the plane was different. Inside the jet, the survivors would stare blankly and then exclaim this was not at all the type of aircraft in which they flew. This was even true for flight attendants and other airline personnel, who thought that the seating arrangement was changed and the position of the interior dividers was unrecognizable. The victims were permitted to relive the flight. They would sit in the exact seat and open the same wing rescue door, crawling on the floor and at times sobbing like children in my arms. The pilot who started the big jet and offered his seat to a survivor to show how cramped his cockpit was and a mechanic who brought a twisted piece of the crashed plane for survivors to smell and touch were both therapists in their own way.

At the time of this writing, an airplane crash in Los Angeles awakened PTSD symptoms in airplane crash survivors all over the world, and I received numerous calls. Each tragedy highlights the victims' personal experiences of their own airplane crash.

After the 1988 airplane crash, similar meetings were again held, provided by the American Red Cross for the volunteers, counselors, ministers, psychologists, and social workers. A yearly update for disas-ter workers is now being implemented, with life support training for physicians. A day-long seminar with experiences and a nationally featured speaker is being planned for those seeking recertification as disaster workers.

Libidinal Cocoon Revisited: Guadalupe River Drownings

The Dallas community suffered another catastrophe July 18, 1987, when a church camp bus was swept away by the Guadalupe River. Ten children drowned, and 33 survivors again were responded to by members of the Texas Psychiatric Society. The small Baptist church in East Dallas sponsored its own libidinal cocoon to take care of its own members, excluding most professional caregivers because of religious concerns.

I was contacted by the media within an hour of the disaster to see what psychiatric services might be provided. This became an opportunity to investigate how group loss and grief could be ministered to by a homogeneous religious unit. The congregation formed a natural libidinal cocoon, allowing the regressive response to loss and grief, with protection from intrusions from the press and the outside world. Members of the congregation took time off from work to meet the needs of their fellow congregants. The church was staffed almost around the clock, much like the hotel used in the airplane crashes. A small police force consisting of four cars and eight officers was stationed on the premises to protect and serve the church.

When I presented myself to the leaders of the church, I felt it important to use counseling within the scriptural framework of that religion, although I was concerned that religious teachings could prevent full expression of the anger that needed to surface in the coming weeks. The elders, deacons, and Sunday-school teachers developed a model that we used as survivors and families of lost children returned from the river site.

The children experienced little specific physical trauma other than a few cases of fractured ribs, several cases of infection, and bruises and sprains. The American Red Cross nurse disaster team assigned a nurse to each family that experienced a loss. As in the past, a Red Cross nurse trained in disaster work proved invaluable.

PTSD was evident in the children as well as in the families. Some refused to participate directly in the groups we established but would cling instead to the fringes, tearful and withdrawn. On several occasions, the families requested that I make house calls to particularly distressed individuals. I noted the families and children participated in their religion in their homes as fervently as they did at the church services. Only one family who lost a child did not fully participate in the services and work of catharsis. The many funeral services, which lasted 2 or more hours, facilitated the group process of grieving.

During the 3 years after the disaster, the parents who lost one or two children were seen on an ongoing basis. The surviving siblings, ranging in age from 13 to 18, were treated in psychotherapy individually or in groups according to their need. A community-level libidinal cocoon assisted the therapeutic regression of the children and families to deal with the loss and grief within the Baptist doctrine. The community allowed me to enter their cocoon, even letting me ride in the limousines with families to funeral services. Surely this was a reaffirmation of the importance of the role of the caring family physician.

Fundamental Protestant religions encourage a variety of practices that fit well into disaster work (Naisbitt and Aburdene 1990). "Witnessing" or confessing before God and the congregation one's shortcomings allows emotional catharsis and permits the laying on of hands physically to console a victim. The concept of Grace allows a belief in forgiveness from God for any and all sins, such as letting go of a good friend's hand who subsequently drowned in the flood. Although an altar call on national television during a funeral in which six caskets are open may not be palatable to many, the congregants were grateful to bring their evangelism nationwide. The charismatic leaders of the Church and the schoolteachers in the adjacent religious school quickly grasped a few fundamentals from me to enhance their own libidinal cocoon by using their own "spiritual gifts." The children were taught that God entered their lives that fateful day and that they were stronger for it.

> A teenage boy with a leukemia and an indwelling peritoneal catheter found himself up a tree while putrid raging waters tore off his wig and infected his wound site. Knowing he was immunocompromised with steroids, he "offered himself up to God." When he was finally rescued after 4 hours in the water, he simply smiled as we put massive amounts of antibiotics inside him. He said his religion had given him an inner peace and he did not need anxiolytics.

A very athletic male had a frail younger girl pulled out of his hands. In a series of dreams he worked through the traumatic event. In his early dreams he dreamt that he had a pole the doomed girl held on to. A few months later he dreamt that he and the girl were sitting on the bank watching the raging flood. In his final dreams they sat together watching the scene on television. His dreams distanced himself and finally her from the horrible drowning scene, and a year later he dreamt of the two of them watching a placid body of water together.

Finally, these young people made direct career choices that reflected their working through of the trauma. Some became water safety instructors; others chose to study civil engineering to learn to build dams to control the elements that almost destroyed them. The teachers taught their classes at times with tears in their eyes and left empty seats unfilled in the tiny classrooms. In school classes, they would readily interrupt a lecture to comment on a theme of loss or to offer a prayer for one of the fallen children. From studying rivers in Texas to studying drowning in first aid and physical education, the congregation and school single-mindedly set about to minister to each other.

Aftermath of Hurricane Hugo in St. Croix

The urgent call from the American Red Cross asked me to report to a briefing in 4 hours at the American Red Cross headquarters. Days before, Hurricane Hugo had devastated the Virgin Islands in the Caribbean and was headed toward South Carolina. The statistics were grim. On St. Croix 96% of the entire island was decimated; St. Thomas was damaged to a lesser degree. The American Red Cross dispatched a group consisting of two psychologists, two social workers, a Red Cross worker, and me to provide aid in Puerto Rico.

The stench of stale urine and feces overwhelmed the flight crew when the aircraft door was opened in San Juan. The heat and odors caused most people to step back in the plane before staggering out into another world. The whole city was paralyzed. Teams of rescue workers were met by troops stationed all along the highways; running water was unavailable, and electrical power was almost nonexistent. Uprooted trees and power lines crisscrossed the wide boulevards. Long lines formed of people awaiting food and staples.

At the Coast Guard station the next morning a brief lecture on survival was given. Hordes of volunteers were separated into groups to match their skills with the needs of the outer islands. My first task was to assess the physical handicaps of volunteers. A typical Red Cross volunteer was often a middle-aged, retired person with a desire to help. Checking vital signs of the volunteers often led to the discovery of the need for multiple medications, usually targeting cardiovascular illness, despite the fact that every health form had "no medical illness" or "no medications" checked. It would have been wise to have required volunteers to have physical examinations and certification of good health before departing. Several people in poor health were sent back protesting loudly. Although loyal and hardworking, they did not realize that their 3 weeks of medication were not going to be enough to carry them through; no medications were available on the islands as the pharmacies had been looted or were under water.

As we flew over the island, the countryside below looked as if a large feather pillow had opened, leaving bits of white fluff (houses and hotels) scattered at random below. We were to find that not a piece of straight tin or a board was left intact on the island. After landing, I went to the Red Cross headquarters to meet with the other physicians on the island. The two physicians already there were buried under lines of patients that never seemed to shorten by day or night. The major hospital had been irreparably damaged, and the Army had set up a tent city outside for generators and potable water supplies. Food packets were being passed out to a hostile, dependent population. At night United States marshals enforced a curfew and martial law to prevent violence and looting.

As has been noted at other disasters, psychosis seemed to yield temporarily to the reality principle, and surprisingly little antipsychotic medication was required. One schizophrenic patient who walked off a building stopped hallucinating immediately as emergency medical care was initiated. Later he and other ambulatory psychotic patients in St. Croix were reestablished on their maintenance antipsychotic medications.

In working with the American Red Cross and island nurses it became evident that basic medical skills were sorely needed, and I was transformed into a general practitioner with psychiatric expertise. The total lack of electricity made it impossible to use a microscope, an incubator, or a hemodialysis unit. Rather, we were preoccupied by problems such as procuring or substituting medications. Although making rounds in school gymnasiums is not a unique experience, rounds with a military squad with armed AR15s was unusual. Outlying schools were converted into large holding areas with rows of bunks or pallets in each room. Ill patients were placed to one side and ministered to by families or community volunteers. As tropical climate conditions prevailed without air conditioning or running water, dysentery and other infectious diseases emerged as causes of illness and death. Garbage piled up, attracting rats and other scavengers. Once-friendly pets became vicious and attacked their former owners or passersby.

Very few psychiatric medications were initially used. Rather, the most important task initially was to visit each holding area and school and attend to medical needs. Other physicians on the island were helped by the military medics and corpsmen. While initially the death rate was low, caregivers soon began to show signs of stress.

The descent of middle-aged and older volunteers from all over the United States on islands designed for vacations and high living created culture shock for both volunteers and the local population. Some volunteers became less functional; others seemed to function on nervous energy alone. After a few days many experienced malaise and global depression as they felt overwhelmed by the task they faced. Every day long lists of essential supplies were requested from the mainland, but the next day's planes delivered items that were neither requested nor needed. As medications taken from the mainland began to run out, other supplies were unnecessarily hoarded. Caregivers began to quarrel among themselves, and daily briefings became like group therapy sessions. The islanders became increasingly hostile, asking questions for which we did not have answers. The military began to accompany us, as if we were dangerous people ourselves. At times, all work would stop when American politicians and officials paraded through the area, surrounded by a phalanx of soldiers bristling with automatic weapons. As the sun set at night, the United States marshals would start tight patrols. Caregivers, even with a large Red Cross insignia, were in danger if they became isolated outside the perimeter of these secured areas.

In retrospect there were certain fundamental truths to be gleaned from such an experience. In times of severe stress people with chronic mental illness seem to rise to the occasion and function at a higher level. The paranoid patients say, "I told you so," and become temporarily part of the human race. The somatoform invalid and anxious patients rally for the moment. Even the depressed patients were able to reach temporarily outside their melancholy selves and render care to others. This respite, however, could be measured in hours or days. By the fourth day after the hurricane, predisaster symptoms returned.

St. Croix and other island disasters have certain elements in common that distinguish them from the mainland. Because an island has discrete boundaries, supply lines are invariably by sea or air. Small islands with no natural resources are particularly vulnerable to isolation without access to basic life supplies. When medical supplies are destroyed, hoarding, stockpiling, and often looting occur unless prevented by law enforcement. Caregivers are perceived as "haves" while the population experiences itself as the "have nots." A sullen anger in the native Crucian population on St. Croix made the delivery of medical and psychiatric services more difficult.

A physician may impart a sense of calm and caring. Many times I rode in the jeep and walked through a large triage area with a smile and a stethoscope and a prayer, having long since run out of medications and bandages. The nurses frequently were thankful for my presence, and I tried to offer support and encouragement. As I rode to the next school or catchment area my own tears reflected the sadness of despair around me. Much of what I did was listen and absorb.

Perhaps the sense of being a leader of a medical team and the knowledge that I could soon leave helped me not to feel overwhelmed. As island physicians presented cases to me, I sensed that my support and encouragement were more important than concrete advice. These were not formal rounds with formal psychiatric examinations but crisis intervention as hordes of problems cascaded on us. The United States seemed very far away.

Conclusions

A unique aspect of airplane crashes is that victims may have little or no connection with the crash site community. In effect the city or region is a "host" for bereavement and often the repository of much anger and hostility. A goal of mental health workers at the crash site community may be to prevent further traumatization in the acute phase and to encourage further therapy after the victim returns home. Notably, after the Dallas airplane crashes, many survivors returned to Dallas for therapy, feeling that city was the appropriate place to do some type of behavioral modification.

A different situation existed after the Guadalupe River drownings. Victims experienced tragedy within their community and continued to live in proximity to the origin of their traumatic experience. The small Baptist church was in a working-class community of blue-collar workers for whom religion was an integral part of daily life. Their fundamentalist religion depicts the struggle of humans with the environment as an overwhelming adversarial conflict, with the forces of evil or judgment ever-present; this provided a framework for shaping the victims' understanding of the tragedy. If this had been an Episcopal, Lutheran, or Unitarian congregation, the working-through phases may have been more difficult. The very conservative and concrete translation of the Bible supplied a precedent for suffering and pain, and the notion that pain leads to ultimate salvation and Grace (i.e., "stars in my crown").

The St. Croix experience was unique in that the island was totally devastated without available reservoirs of assistance, geographically or financially. The native population had no source of income or skills to help themselves. With a history of dependence on agencies or governmental assistance, they became easily overwhelmed by their inability to provide themselves with food, clothing, or shelter. Their dependency fostered hostility; rioting and pillaging captured national headlines, which ostracized and further isolated them. The military presence changed the character of the caregivers' attitudes by the creation of a war zone mentality. This was underscored by the curfew, as the dangers for the health teams were always a paramount consideration.

What do these experiences imply about the psyche of the caregiver? I relied heavily on my two very orthodox analytic experiences dealing with losses early in my life to explain my interest in the bereavement process in my practice and my volunteer work. With loss comes anger, often directed at those in power. This is followed by a search for answers, the introspective "Why?" Experiences of life, death, and tragedy impel us to explain how we got here, what our goals are, and where we expect to go in an afterlife, if anywhere.

Disaster experiences reignite the universal wish of people to be taken care of, despite (or because of) the marginal nature of the childhood experience for many. The extended morbidity for some victims reflects the precarious underpinnings of their developmental stages and the difficulty resolving the strong regressive pull of infantilization versus the need to resume adult living and to go on with their lives and responsibilities.

There are basically two requirements for psychological growth. The first condition to be satisfied is that the individual has mastered the tasks of the present level and is comfortable in extending or stretching a bit to take on the next level. The second condition is that the next level is not too threatening or formidable to negotiate. Many people who are capable of presenting a superficial appearance of normalcy have weak ego structures. These people may fit into the borderline personality category and may readily regress or become temporarily psychotic under stressful conditions. Thus disasters, with their massive stressors, may unmask latent defects in personalities that were not seen before the trauma.

Many of the above individuals will drift into some kind of therapy or religion or both in an attempt to mend their fragmented childhood experiences; needy patients may almost "enjoy" the regression after a trauma and be very slow to reconstitute and regain their previously unpalatable and unrewarded state in life. The therapist will have a fragile alliance with these patients who experience their lives as a "disaster" in which their fantasized needs far outstrip the available assets and thus look to the caregiver to fulfill their perceived deficits (Frank 1968).

Professional caregivers are natural targets for the wish for someone to "make it better." It is a rare caregiver who can maintain therapeutic neutrality in crisis intervention and the recovery, carefully titrating initial gratification and pushing for psychological growth. The therapeutic process will be to withhold gently the regressive elements of therapy when appropriate, while encouraging increasing autonomy.

What type of psychiatrist might work best with a survivor or family member waiting for autopsy reports or dealing with a hospitalized relative? It would seem that the ability of the therapist to tolerate a large amount of regression would be beneficial. Although disaster response activity may seem very different from classic psychoanalytic technique, psychoanalysts are uniquely trained to tolerate and experience empathetically the regressive pull of an individual or group of individuals caught up in a vortex of regressive infantilized behavior. This would also include therapists who are comfortable in dealing with terminal physical illness, such as acquired immunodeficiency syndrome (AIDS) or cancer.

In the initial crisis setting of mass casualty, issues of bonding and transference are of great importance and intensity. The physician who is not able to withstand an onslaught of primitive wishes and who needs gratification measures may be more comfortable visiting patients in a team with other helping professionals. This allows diffusion of the transference to an institution or group rather than to an individual.

Therapists who are trained to interpret rather than gratify transference wishes may take a blank screen stance. The mass casualty victim may experience this as coldly frustrating. Thus, people who may tolerate regression but who are unable to gratify wishes may not do well with mass casualty PTSD patients. Although obviously not all of a patient's wishes should be indiscriminately gratified, nonetheless some indulgence and sector parameters should be considered. For example, the ability to utilize medical skills to examine certain aches or pains may be helpful in some situations, since other physicians may be unavailable. The ability to nurture in a constructive way may help the patient who has regressed to an earlier level, experiencing old frustrations that occurred when powerful figures seemed to withhold help or attention.

Therapists must also be comfortable with their own reaction to carnage and losses in earlier life and be secure in the knowledge that what they are offering in the long run will be beneficial to the family or the patient. A tremendous need surfaces in most therapists to be accepted and "liked." This may be in contradiction to the situation of deprivation and loss. It may well serve the therapist to be able to absorb anger and rage and not feel annihilated and to be able to reassure in a calm manner and go about one's duties in the face of covert or overt hostility, both from victims and from "authorities," such as airline or government officials.

Specific problems may plague health workers responding to the identified psychiatric patient and the patient's family. Often it is difficult to offer support to a potentially stigmatized person who has not had a positive experience with a health caregiver in the past. Other patients may be reluctant to document medication or a psychiatric background for fear of the impact on a potential settlement from an outside agency. Because local newspapers have carried stories of the airlines using survivors' history of psychiatric treatment as a defense in litigation, it is understandable that many families or survivors are reluctant to talk to mental health workers because of feared connections with airlines. The American Red Cross badge is invaluable as a talisman in these cases.

Although medications may at times be helpful, certain precautions should be taken. Benzodiazepines may be useful to treat acute anxiety or insomnia, but may also increase the potential for psychogenic amnesia seen in PTSD (Smith and Juhl 1984). However, if used judiciously with appropriate documentation, major and minor tranquilizers may be useful with minimal effect on memory or performance. After one airplane crash, as I worked with survivors in my office, I was astonished to find that some dozen very educated and healthy young adults gave crash descriptions and drew pictures that were significantly different from each other. The sounds, timing, and geographic position of the plane in its environment during the last 23 seconds of flight were alarmingly dissimilar. By making exact records and not overmedicating PTSD survivors, the caregiver may help diminish the amnestic fugue states that frequently occur (Subhan et al. 1986). The literature shows that once a steady state is achieved with benzodiazepines, there is little effect on memory or performance (Kumar et al. 1987).

General medical skills may be invaluable for the psychiatrist, especially in disaster settings in which the availability of other medical personnel may be limited. These skills are especially helpful in ministering to elderly patients, whose predisaster medical status may have been precarious. The psychiatrist may need to triage such patients for further treatment by other specialists.

The team leader should attempt to exude confidence to the team and set an example of communicating warmth and understanding to victims. Perhaps the most valuable gift is the one of empathic understanding and acceptance of human frailties and culpability. The ultimate goal is to be truly "with" a traumatized family in their moment of greatest need. Supportive care and education during the most acute phase may ease the transfer of patients back to their local caregivers and supportive institutions.

References

American Psychiatric Association: Diagnostic and Statistical Manual of Mental Disorders, 3rd Edition, Revised. Washington, DC, American Psychiatric Association, 1987

American Psychiatric Association: Let's Talk Facts About Post-Traumatic Stress Disorder. Washington, DC, American Psychiatric Association, 1988

Black JW: The libidinal cocoon: a nurturing retreat for the families of plane crash victims. Hosp Community Psychiatry 38:1322–1326, 1987

Frank JD: The influence of patients' and therapists' expectations on the outcome of the psychotherapy. Br J Med Psychol 41:349–356, 1968

Kumar R, Aalijits M, Babrielli W, et al: Anxiolytics and memory: a comparison of lorazepam and alprazolam. J Clin Psychiatry 48:158–160, 1987

Naisbitt J, Aburdene P: Megatrends 2000. New York, Morrow & Co, 1990

Smith RB, Juhl RP: Pharmacokinetics and pharmacodynamics of alprazolam after oral and IV administration. Psychopharmacology 84:452–456, 1984

Subhan Z, Harrison C, Hindmarch I: Alprazolam and lorazepam single and multiple dose effects on psychomotor skills and sleep. Eur J Clin Pharmacol 29:709–712, 1986

Additional Readings

Brett EA, Ostroff R: Imagery and posttraumatic stress disorder: an overview. Am J Psychiatry 142:417–424, 1985

Davanloo H: Basic Principles and Techniques in Short-Term Dynamic Psychotherapy. New York, Spectrum, 1978

Lindemann E: Symptomatology and management of acute grief. Am J Psychiatry 101:141–148, 1944

Malan DH: A Study of Brief Psychotherapy. London, Tavistock, 1963

Ott J: Women Viet Nam veterans, in The Trauma of War: Stress and Recovery in Viet Nam Veterans. Edited by Sonnenberg SM, Blank AS, Talbott JA. Washington, DC, American Psychiatric Press, 1985, pp 137–157

Pynoos R, Nader K: Psychological first aid and treatment approach to children exposed to community violence: research implications. Journal of Traumatic Stress 1:445–473, 1988

Rubin H: The American Psychiatric Association Clergy Packet. Washington, DC, American Psychiatric Association, 1989

Sifneos PE: Short-Term Dynamic Psychotherapy. New York, Spectrum, 1978

Wilkinson CB: Aftermath of a disaster: the collapse of the Hyatt Regency Hotel skywalks. Am J Psychiatry 140:1134–1139, 1983

Chapter 11

Function of Mobile Crisis Intervention Teams After Hurricane Hugo

Joseph J. Zealberg, M.D.
Jackie Puckett, A.C.S.W.

I have seen tempests when the scolding winds have rived the knotty oaks, and I have seen th' ambitious ocean swell and rage and foam to be exalted with the threat'ning clouds.

William Shakespeare

*O*n September 21, 1989, fear crept into the hearts of hundreds of thousands of Americans living on the southeastern coast of the United States as Hurricane Hugo rapidly approached. The storm had wrought a path of destruction as it crossed the Virgin Islands and Puerto Rico, leaving billions of dollars in damages as it continued its northwestern journey toward the American mainland. In this chapter we focus on the role of our emergency psychiatry/mobile crisis team and its response to the most destructive natural disaster in the history of the United States.

The emergency team normally functions as the collaborative psychiatric emergency service for the Charleston Area Mental Health Center and the Medical University of South Carolina. The program's clinical staff is thoroughly experienced in dealing with severe psychiatric emergencies, both in emergency rooms and in the community at large. However, no one living in the Charleston area had ever witnessed a storm of such intensity. The crisis team had been given the responsibility for coordinating emergency mental health disaster services for Charleston County, and this was their first experience with a disaster of this type.

Preimpact Phase

On September 20, the citizens of South Carolina's coastal areas were ordered by government officials to evacuate. Crisis services' staffs were instructed to evacuate for safety and to contact the directors by beeper as soon as the storm passed. Although most of Charleston's inhabitants evacuated, the directors of the emergency psychiatry service felt that it was necessary to remain in the community so that mental health services could be coordinated and delivered throughout all phases of the storm. The emergency services program manager (J. P.) coordinated activities with civil defense authorities at the Emergency Operations Center. The program director (J. Z.) went to a local high school, which had been converted to a hurricane shelter housing approximately 500 people. Both of the program's emergency automobiles were parked on high ground areas believed to be safe, and the emergency psychopharmacologic drug boxes and cellular telephones were locked away at the hurricane shelter. As time quickly passed, it became clear that landfall for Hurricane Hugo would be directly over Charleston.

After arriving at the high school shelter, the emergency psychiatric director communicated with shelter officials and consulted with the principal, who was in charge. Several hours before the storm arrived, the principal was advised to gather everyone to give them an idea of what was to come. The shelter plan was designed to have lights out by a certain time that evening, since it was readily apparent that a category 4 storm would clearly knock out all utility power. People were instructed to prepare their flashlights ahead of time and to expect to hear deafening amounts of noise, wind, sounds of rushing, roaring, and sounds similar to "freight trains" all around the shelter. Volunteers from within the shelter were instructed to circulate throughout the shelter complex and constantly reassure people that things would be fine and to remain calm. Provisions were made to evacuate efficiently the shelter inhabitants from the first to the second floor in the event of a storm surge flood.

As Hurricane Hugo approached landfall, satellite pictures indicated that the storm itself was probably larger than the entire state of South Carolina, which has an area of 30,207 square miles. All local television and radio communications were suddenly silenced by the 135 mph winds.

Impact Phase

As the storm passed over the area, there was a strange and eerie silence within the high school shelter. The wind sounded like battering rams against the doors and windows. High-pitched snapping sounds were heard often; the next morning, it became clear that this was the sound of large trees being instantaneously broken in half by the wind. Backup generators "died," windows and roofs were blown off, and many people feared for their lives. It quickly became evident that a person would be unlikely to understand the psychological trauma caused by a hurricane without living through one. Volunteers in the shelters were able to identify people who were suffering from acute, severe emotional trauma and would ask for those persons to be evaluated further.

> A young mother of three children spent 2 days in the shelter prior to the hurricane. About 10 minutes after the ferocious storm struck, a look of terror and anxiety was evident in her dazed expression. A volunteer noticed that she had begun to rock back and forth, while repeating "is it over, is it over," even though she "knew" the hurricane would last several hours. Because of her great fear, she required constant reassurance that the storm was indeed "almost over." This repeated, quiet reassurance helped prevent her from losing control of herself.
>
> During the eye of the hurricane, a young man began screaming for hundreds of people to leave the shelter. He said he was "in charge," and everyone should leave their garbage "for him." The man was clearly hypomanic and grandiose, and intervention was immediately begun, including redirecting him to his family, giving verbal reassurance that we were all going to live through the storm, and administering benzodiazepines as needed. He was then able to remain calm with his family during the latter half of the storm.

The next morning one person said she fantasized that the storm was the devil looking for victims. She said that she knew if she made any noise or if anyone in the room made any noise that "he" (the devil) would know that we were within, and "he" would break down the windows and doors and kill everyone. Numerous people used a similar metaphor and said that having volunteers available to walk around and reassure the evacuees in the shelter helped them cope with extreme fear.

As the storm passed, some 6 hours later, contact was initiated via telephone with the state's central Emergency Operations Center 100 miles away in Columbia, the state's capital. By that time, more than half of the state was without power, a situation that would last for weeks in many areas.

Postimpact Phase

By daylight, the entire Charleston area had changed. Many areas had flooded under the 17-foot tidal surge, and other areas looked as if they had been bombed. Trees blocked sections of roads and cut through houses. Boats were on highways. Virtually every power line and pole was down, causing 750,000 people to be without power. Where forests and woods once stood, broken stumps remained. Approximately 65,000 people in South Carolina were suddenly homeless. Twenty-nine people who had remained in the area died. Thousands would have perished if the evacuation order had not been given. In one night's passing, the entire face of South Carolina had been altered. The devastation was overwhelming. Many areas looked as if they had been bombed. The cost of damages to South Carolina alone was approximately 6 billion dollars.

Few psychiatric emergencies were seen in the next 2 days. After witnessing Hugo's destructive power, most people were in a state of denial and shock, aware of how glad they were to be alive. In the face of such massive destruction, people felt that their most important possessions (i.e., material items, belongings, and personal property) suddenly became less important than basic needs: Am I alive? Do I have food? Do I have water? An awareness of those basic needs softened the pain of the immediate trauma. For example, people would say "I have only lost my house but the guy up the street lost his house, his boat, and his car. I guess I'm really lucky." This change in perspective helped people through traumas that otherwise would have damaged their psychological state of well-being. Many described a form of survivor's guilt, especially those who were less affected by the storm; those individuals, in turn, were able to share their good fortune with others, thus diminishing guilt-induced psychological disequilibrium.

Those in the helping professions realized that they needed to mobilize their services to help the community at large. Due to the lack of transportation, the imposition of curfews, and the overwhelming disorganization the victims experienced, victims were often unable to get to clinics, hospitals, or emergency rooms. Because of these situations, it became necessary to mobilize services within the community at large.

The sense of loss and sadness was obvious in Charlestonians as everywhere one looked, one saw people displaced, homeless, and in psychological shock. The presence of National Guard military units seemed to exaggerate this feeling. Suddenly, the rubble that was in the streets, the homeowners searching through debris, and the military-clad men in the background with fixed bayonets and automatic weapons were not on a newsreel from another country but were present in Charleston, South Carolina. A sense of surrealism exacerbated the anxiety that everyone experienced.

Within a day, the emergency psychiatric team set up a "command post" at the main mental health center building, which had survived the storm (seven of nine mental health center buildings were destroyed, however). Portable cellular telephones and gasoline-powered generators allowed the staff to organize a central communication and treatment center for patients and walk-in emergencies. Thereafter, as radio transmission became available, the director of the mental health center made numerous announcements to notify the public that emergency mental health services were available at the local county hospital emergency department, at the mental health center, and in the community via mobile crisis intervention.

Perhaps one of the most critical components of our disaster plan was the linkage with the central office of the South Carolina Department of Mental Health (SCDMH). Before the storm, the department had arranged for "Go-teams" to be formed from various DMH agencies throughout the state, including community mental health centers and inpatient units. These Go-teams included psychiatric aides, nurses, psychologists, and people with administrative expertise. Those teams rotated every 3–5 days through the hurricane-ravaged areas and were prepared to do whatever was necessary to address the mental health needs of the disaster victims. After briefing, the Go-teams were quickly disbursed to various shelters in the area and were able to begin dealing effectively with shelter residents' mental health and other needs as appropriate.

It was quickly learned that, in the face of a disaster, one's usual job description is completely meaningless. At first, there was little coordination of services. For example, our psychiatric emergency service had to deal with many of the medical problems that patients were experiencing as there was little coordinated effort to provide acute medical care in the community. Over time, however, communication linkages were set up, and more appropriate channels were found.

In a disaster everything changes. The real suddenly becomes unreal, and the familiar, unfamiliar. The result is extremely disorienting and anxiety provoking. Familiar places had become almost unrecognizable due to lack of lighting, signs, or other means of obtaining orientation and direction. Food, ice, batteries, and generators were scarce, and water was undrinkable in many areas. Communication after Hugo was at a total standstill. We found that the use of cellular telephones in our automobiles was invaluable to us. However, there were times when the phones were unusable, and the only way of linking up and communicating with the Emergency Operations Center was to make several car trips per day to coordinate and communicate with those at the center. It was important to centralize the communication facilities so that major needs could be addressed and resources distributed in a coordinated and efficient way.

In addition to the Go-teams, the SCDMH sent teams of two SCDMH public safety officers per 12-hour shift. One guarded our medicine supplies, and the other was available to accompany the mobile crisis team on calls occurring in the Charleston community. Ordinarily, our mobile emergency team asks local law enforcement officers to join them on a call only if necessary. However, after the hurricane, local police were relatively unavailable since they were involved in numerous activities such as traffic control or prevention of criminal activities. The area was placed under martial law, and a curfew was imposed, making the populace very fearful and apprehensive. The armed soldiers of the National Guard began to appear everywhere. The SCDMH police officers allowed us to deal with most psychiatric emergencies in an efficient, safe manner, with minimal anxiety.

Because of a lack of resources and the presence of overwhelming psychological trauma, it quickly became apparent that our mobile outreach capabilities were needed throughout the community. The local emergency rooms were becoming rapidly overcrowded due to the large number of accidental injuries in the community during clean-up efforts after the storm (e.g., chain-saw accidents, cuts from broken glass or nails, fractures caused by falls, and traffic-related injuries due to the absence of electricity and traffic signals). We therefore decided to treat as many people as possible at their home or shelter. As the official civil defense coordinators for emergency mental health care, we were able to travel through restricted areas in an unencumbered fashion and could also network with other systems for badly needed supplies, such as food, water, and medicines.

As the emergency service responded to community calls, the most helpful initial interventions involved supportive listening. Each person seen in crisis had a unique and often heroic story to tell.

> A law enforcement officer narrowly escaped death in a storm surge flood and was unable to decrease his state of fear and anxiety. An emergency psychiatrist met with him and allowed him to retell the frightening experience of almost drowning in the tidal surge and the extreme guilt he felt at being unable to provide for the safety of others caught in the flooding storm shelter. Fortunately, no one was seriously injured, and the officer was reassured that he did everything possible to preserve the life of those around him. He was given several tablets of lorazepam and was allowed to leave duty for a few days on our advice. After several days he returned to duty. This immediate intervention may have diminished the likelihood of his anxiety evolving into a complete, sustained posttraumatic stress disorder.

> A man with schizophrenia was seen for exacerbation of psychosis. He had stayed in his home during the hurricane while his house was destroyed around him. He appeared to be in a state of emotional shock and said he "couldn't stand the voices." We listened to him and gave him something to drink (bottled water, a precious commodity), some haloperidol, and a few hugs. After 2 hours he felt better. Two days later our team happened to see him at the busiest public shelter, where he had been volunteering to help others. He smiled and asked, "Remember me?"

Traditional lines of professional practice had to be blurred at times. Often, primary care responsibilities had to be dealt with before psychiatric intervention.

> Numerous indigent people were in shelters, lacking medications for chronic medical conditions, such as epilepsy, diabetes, and severe hypertension. A psychiatry professor who volunteered to help the mobile team spent several hours on the phone with numerous agencies in an effort to procure emergency medical supplies. His energetic

efforts allowed many medically ill people to restart treatment with insulin, antihypertensives, anticonvulsants, and other medicines.

Because of the severe shortage of alcoholic beverages, many substance-dependent people began to present for emergency evaluation of alcohol withdrawal.

> A woman made homeless by Hugo was seen at a shelter 1 week after the storm. She had stayed in her beachfront home during the hurricane, clutching her dog in an upstairs closet while the wind and waves destroyed most of her beach house around her. The following day she went on a whiskey-drinking binge that lasted 3 days. On examination, we found her to be in alcohol withdrawal delirium, complicated by severe pancreatitis. We referred her to an internal medicine ward for emergency treatment.

In addition to seeing acute psychiatric and medical crises within the community, we would occasionally have to assist psychiatrically ill people from out of town who came to Charleston to assist in relief efforts.

> A manic woman from another state came to Charleston to "do God's work and help everyone in need." We were called to see her because she was trying to take over a shelter's operation. Unfortunately, her mania caused her to be hospitalized.

Suicide calls were common in the weeks after the storm.

> A former naval officer was washed out of his bed when the storm surge broke through his windows. For several weeks he had increasing anxiety and depressive symptoms with nightmares. He called the mobile team in an intoxicated, suicidal state with a loaded revolver in his hand. The team arrived at his home, talked him into relinquishing the gun, and hospitalized him.

The emergency psychiatry team not only treated primary victims, but helping professionals too.

> A nurse who volunteered at one of the public shelters quickly became overwhelmed by the sight of several hundred homeless individuals, many of whom had lost their life's possessions. The nurse began to cry, saying, "I can't be here! I can't take it!" Our clinical staff were able to

talk with her and support her ego defenses. In a short time, she had regained her composure and effectively completed her work at the shelter.

Discussion

In the wake of a natural disaster, people experience a numbness of thinking that is extremely disorienting. This affects disaster relief workers who may be victims, too. The breadth of destruction after Hugo changed the cognitive-perceptual map of Charlestonians overnight. Because of the associated anxiety and disorganization, it was difficult to organize disaster relief systems; the existence of an emergency plan was therefore critical. Everyone in the local mental health center agreed that the emergency psychiatric service would take initial coordination leadership in the event of disaster, and we had full administrative support for this responsibility. After emergency mental health services were set up and coordinated, administrative leadership was returned to those normally in charge. Normal institutional working operations were reintroduced over a period of weeks, and the emergency service gradually and naturally returned to its primary focus.

The emergency team constantly interacted with community leaders, media, members of law enforcement, social services, and other agencies. Disaster victims were deprived of vital information, and effective networking on behalf of victims frequently resolved numerous psychiatric crises.

Although the emergency team was able to resolve most crises, little provision or time existed for proper debriefing of the emergency psychiatric clinicians themselves. For example, many clinical staff worked daily for 3 weeks or more without a day off. Normal time cues were absent due to lack of electricity, lighting, and so on, and this, in part, contributed to the rapid passage of time, which almost went unnoticed. Clearly, provisions for proper "time-out" intervals and debriefing sessions should be included for emergency services staff in our future disaster planning. It is extremely difficult to absorb the psychological trauma of disaster victims when one is also a victim.

During times of disaster, numerous community organizations need to work together to respond to the overwhelming physical and psychological trauma that results before, during, and after catastrophes. It is important to have disaster preparedness plans so that numerous community agencies can organize quickly and work cooperatively. Police, fire departments, emergency medical services, and military officials, as well as county, state, and federal systems, need to integrate and work in a coordinated fashion to deliver immediate services to those most in need. Emergency mental health services are important in the development of disaster planning, so that immediate mental health interventions can be provided.

Appropriate mental health leadership involving administrative support is a key element. Early visibility and early interventions are of critical importance. It is important to disseminate mental health information to the public and to provide assertive outreach to disaster victims. This appears to be particularly appropriate for those experiencing psychiatric emergencies. After the Hugo disaster, psychiatrically ill people responded extremely well to relatively little support. With a hug, a dose of psychopharmacologic medicine, some hot coffee, and a few words of encouragement, some patients with severe psychiatric illnesses were able to achieve a rapid state of remission. We often were impressed by the resiliency of the victims.

The experiences of the emergency psychiatry/mobile crisis team during Hugo and its aftermath validate much of the mental health literature on disasters. It has been reported that fear, anxiety, and extreme tension are often found among survivors of numerous types of disasters, such as tornadoes, nuclear plant accidents, earthquakes, train wrecks, floods, and hurricanes (Bates et al. 1963). In addition to anxiety symptoms, depression symptoms and grief reactions frequently occur as well. Survival guilt also occurs frequently, adding to distress of disaster survivors (Lifton and Olson 1976; Tichener and Kapp 1976). Indeed, all of these emotional responses were evident among Hugo's victims.

Of all the disaster-related impacts considered, it seems to be that the direct experience of extreme life-threatening terror and horror is most associated with the development of mental health crises and problems. According to Bolin (1986), terror is most likely to occur in an intense unpredicted disaster, such as flash floods, severe earthquakes, tornadoes, and other experiences in which the disaster agent possesses extreme physical force that the victim directly witnesses or experiences. More than terror, horror is produced by the witnessing of death and the accidental discovery of bodies, seeing the unsightly physical condition of corpses and the nature of causes of death. Such experiences are extremely likely to generate serious mental health problems. Fortunately, in the case of Hugo, due to expert planning, direction, and evacuation notices, horror was kept to an absolute minimum, and few people remained to experience the terror of the storm.

Bolin (1986) also noted that the duration of the impact of the disaster agent may also have a profound effect on its victims. High-intensity, short-duration disasters seem most commonly associated with psychological disturbances. Generally speaking, it appears that major disasters with little or no warning are expected to produce higher levels of psychological stress than those with a long forewarning. It is felt that disasters that are preceded by a warning period of hours to days, such as hurricanes, may not be associated with significant psychological impairment unless the intensity of the agent is such that the impact is very high (Bates et al. 1963). Bolin suggested that the impact ratio, which is the ratio of total loss to available surviving resources, is an important variable in assessing the degree of stress on disaster survivors. This ratio can be viewed in a sense as the proportion of affected to nonaffected community. When impact ratios are low (e.g., when a tornado destroys a small section of a large area), victims can evacuate and remove themselves from the physical effects of the disaster, thus reducing their stress. Obviously, this was not so for Hurricane Hugo, which had such a wide area of destruction. Bolin noted that large-scale disasters are most likely to disrupt an individual's sense of control, particularly those disasters with a high impact ratio and intensity of impact. These effects may create a "nameless feeling that something has gone awry in the order of things . . . that the world as the survivors knew it had come to an end" (Erickson 1976, p. 159). As one Hugo victim commented, "I remember that Friday night after the hurricane. All the lights were out and it felt like all the lights in the world were gone."

Quarantelli and Dynes (1973) summarized community effects and responses in the aftermath of a disaster. In communities, an emergency consensus forms following a disaster, and altruistic norms emerge. They believe that negative mental health consequences most likely occur when community priorities are not met in the aftermath of a disaster. Specifically, locating and caring for victims and restoration and maintenance of essential community services, such as utilities, transportation, and communication facilities, are of utmost importance; maintenance of public order and sustaining public morale are also necessary to reintegrate the community and diminish the severe mental health effects on individuals.

Bolin (1986) underscored the idea that communities are complex social entities that constitute symbolic objects of orientation for their residents and are the basis of cognitive maps for people who inhabit such communities. These mental maps render the local community familiar, safe, and readily accessible to its inhabitants. In addition, Hunter (1974) believed communities provide symbolic identification and become part of the residents' personal identities. When these cognitive and social frames become extremely disrupted, as in the aftermath of a disaster, such disruption evokes psychological pain and disorganization in those affected. Because of massive, widespread destruction, Charlestonians were left in a daze, which for many lasted several months.

Tichener and Kapp (1976) reported that during the first days and weeks after the Buffalo Creek Dam flood, which occurred in February 1972 in Buffalo Creek, West Virginia, survivors reported disorganization and sluggishness in their thinking and decision making. In addition, they complained of having difficulty controlling their emotions. These difficulties ranged from emotional lability to emotional numbing. Almost all reported anxiety, grief, and despair, with sleep disturbances and nightmares. Later, the anxiety was manifested with obsessions or phobic behaviors concerning water, wind, rain, and any other reminder that the disaster could recur. These phenomena were also seen by us after Hugo.

We focused much of our clinical energies on high-risk groups: elderly individuals who were house- or shelter-bound and those with a previous psychiatric history or recent overwhelming loss. Smith et al. (1990) studied the prevalence of psychiatric disorders in survivors of a jet plane crash into a hotel. Their findings may indicate that the target population at greatest risk for postdisaster psychiatric syndromes is probably those who have preexisting psychiatric disorders. Almost 100% of those in the high-stress-exposure group who had preexisting depressive disorders had recurrence of depression after the disaster. Psychiatric intervention may therefore be particularly important for that group of individuals and for others with a history of a major psychiatric syndrome. Interestingly, Smith et al. found that almost half of those who were exposed to the trauma of the jet crash did not develop a postdisaster disorder. This is an important fact to remember so that disaster workers and clinicians may focus on issues of health rather than illness after a disaster experience. In our work, most people quickly responded to support and crisis therapy. Many of our colleagues believed that a huge surge of people with postdisaster trauma would appear several weeks after Hugo. This did not happen, suggesting that most people, as in Smith et al.'s group, did not develop a severe disorder. This, in turn, may have occurred because of the tremendous support the community of Charleston received from within itself and from other locales.

Shore (1989) reviewed some of the knowledge regarding psychiatric consequences of disasters. Besides natural disasters, he noted that many people's lives have been affected by airline crashes, kidnappings, terrorist acts, nuclear mishaps, and fears of other such events. In addition, new attention has been focused on the consequences of military stress after the Vietnam War, and more research is being undertaken regarding posttraumatic stress disorder. An understanding of posttraumatic stress disorder stems in part from analyses of people who have survived such disasters as the Boston Coconut Grove nightclub fire, in November 1982 (Lindemann 1944), the Buffalo Creek flood, and the bombing of Hiroshima. More recently, studies were made after the July 1976 Chowchilla, California, kidnapping (Terr 1983); Mount Saint Helens, in Washington State in 1980 (Shore et al. 1986); and Three Mile Island, in Pennsylvania in 1979 (Baum et al. 1983).

Shore (1989) noted that there are two predominant interpretations in the field of disaster research. The first interpretation emphasizes a social view: that is, a disruption of interpersonal and social linkages and the importance of the social support system to determine disaster response. The second view defines the extent to which disaster victims suffer from significant psychiatric disorders as a result of disaster stress. We found that it was necessary to attend to both factors in our post-Hugo crisis intervention. Often, finding social resources for people quickly calmed severe emotional symptoms. The quick action of community leaders and the mutual support from other communities allowed hope to prevail, thus preventing further trauma.

Kinston and Rosser (1974, p. 448) noted that "there is evidence that specialized psychiatric skills could be useful in all phases of a disaster. However, psychiatrists are rarely called upon and their intervention is actively resisted in the early phases by other helpers and in the late phases by the victims themselves." Our experience validated only the first part of their statement. Because of our assertive approach to psychiatric emergencies, and our previous experience in working as a mobile emergency unit within the community, we found our services were utilized completely throughout all phases of the Hurricane Hugo disaster.

After a hurricane or other severe natural disaster, it is important for mental health professionals to mobilize their services within the community. The immediate needs for crisis intervention are apparent, however, only if crisis teams venture out in the immediate disaster areas. If one remains in the office, hospital, or clinic, a false impression may form that few psychiatric crises are occurring. We advocate that an assertive, outreach approach to crisis intervention is always indicated following a major disaster and that emergency psychiatric clinicians should assume leadership roles at these most difficult times of human suffering.

References

Bates FL, Fogelman CW, Partenon VJ, et al: The social and psychological consequences of a natural disaster: a longitudinal study of Hurricane Audrey (Disaster Study 18). Washington, DC, National Academy of Sciences National Research Council, 1963

Baum A, Gatchel RJ, Schaeffer MA: Emotional, behavioral, and physiological effects of chronic stress at Three Mile Island. J Consult Clin Psychol 51:565–572, 1983

Bolin R: Disaster characteristics and psychosocial impacts, in Disasters and Mental Health, Contemporary Perspectives and Innovative Services to Disaster Victims. Edited by Sowder BJ, Lystad M. Washington, DC, American Psychiatric Association, 1986, pp 11–35

Erickson KT: Everything in Its Path: Destruction in the Community in the Buffalo Creek Flood. New York, Simon & Schuster, 1976

Hunter A: Symbolic Communities. Chicago, IL, University of Chicago Press, 1974

Kinston W, Rosser K: Disaster: effects on mental and physical state. J Psychosom Res 19:437–456, 1974

Lifton RJ, Olson E: The human meaning of total disaster: the Buffalo Creek experience. Psychiatry 39:1–18, 1976

Lindemann E: Symptomatology and management of acute grief. Am J Psychiatry 101:141–148, 1944

Quarantelli EL, Dynes RR: Images of Disaster: Myths and Consequences. Columbus, OH, Disaster Relief Center, Ohio State University, 1973

Shore JH: Recent disasters renew interest in PTSD. The Psychiatric Times 6(12):62, 1989

Shore JH, Tatum EL, Vollmer WM: Psychiatric reactions to disaster: the Mount St. Helens experience. Am J Psychiatry 243:590–595, 1986

Smith EM, North CS, McCool RE, et al: Acute post-disaster psychiatric disorders: identification of persons at risk. Am J Psychiatry 147:202–206, 1990

Terr L: Chowchilla revisited: the effects of psychic trauma four years after a school-bus kidnapping. Am J Psychiatry 140:1543–1550, 1983

Tichener JL, Kapp FT: Family and character change at Buffalo Creek. Am J Psychiatry 133:295–299, 1976

Chapter 12

Management of a Psychiatric Inpatient Service During and After Hurricane Hugo

George W. Arana, M.D.
Elizabeth Huggins, R.N., Ph.D.
Hal Currey, B.S.

Approximately 1 week before landfall of Hurricane Hugo, on September 21, 1989, the Medical University of South Carolina (MUSC) Disaster Service began to track the hurricane as it moved through the Caribbean. The disaster control officer held daily meetings with critical members of administration, nursing, and the medical director of the MUSC Medical Center to apprise them of the direction, speed, and intensity of the hurricane. As the hurricane neared the mainland, 72 hours before actual landfall, the risk of a direct hit to Charleston, South Carolina, was evaluated as an increasing probability. At this time the medical director of the psychiatric facility began to attend the MUSC disaster control team meetings and served as a communications link between the university and the facility. The executive management team began to review general plans for handling the potential disaster within the psychiatric facility, and preparation for the disaster was begun.

Effectively coping with the problems of a natural disaster within a medical facility may be related to the management structure in place before the disaster. We believe that the success in managing the Hugo disaster in our institution was the product of a team approach philosophy that was already in operation. The framework developed by the team was based on communication, planning, and flexibility (Table 12–1). The hospital executive team is composed of the medical director

(G.W.A.), the director of inpatient nursing (E.H.), and the hospital administrator (H.C.). These individuals work together as a nonhierarchical team. This same structure is reflected at the unit level, with the physician and nurse in partnership serving as unit coordinator. At the time of the storm, the executive team and unit coordinators were meeting weekly to oversee the operation of the Institute of Psychiatry and to serve as a communications link between the units and the executive team. This structure served us well before, during, and after the storm.

The psychiatric facility is a three-story, acute-care hospital with two floors for adult psychiatric inpatients and one floor for child and adolescent patients. Each floor is operated as a separate unit with its own physician and nurse-coordinator team. The hospital executive team decided to convene a meeting with all the unit coordinators to begin specific planning and decision making for the increasing probability that Hurricane Hugo would strike Charleston. This group met twice daily for the next 7 days.

By the time Hugo was within 24 hours of Charleston, a plan was in effect to discharge all stable patients who were able to leave the facility. Also, in the 12 hours before landfall of Hugo, a contingency plan was developed to evacuate the entire first floor of the facility in case extreme flooding developed. Communications plans were also developed so that rapid communications could take place with the staff to cope with critical planning changes that were anticipated.

Table 12–1.   Framework for disaster management

Communication	Planning	Flexibility
1. Twice-daily meeting with management staff	1. Twice-daily meeting	1. Staff housing
2. Management availability	2. Task assignment	2. Child care
3. Daily meeting with entire staff	3. Patient rounds	3. Adjustment in administrative roles
	4. Staff groups	4. Staff groups
		5. Delay in admission
		6. After-storm groups

The following is a detailed description of how the three administrative sections of the MUSC Institute of Psychiatry responded to Hugo.

Physical Plant Administration

Disaster Planning

In the meetings with the MUSC disaster control team, the supply of critical items, such as electrical power, water, and food, was discussed in detail. Although potential problems were explored at length, the water supply company assured the hospital that the water supply could not become a problem because a new and updated system had been installed and that they were ready for any possible disaster. It was also anticipated that the electrical power would not be jeopardized since the hospital had its own generators to power critical areas within the facility. The psychiatric facility also had its own recently tested generator to provide power. Since the psychiatric facility is freestanding and relatively remote from the main hospital, any flooding would cut off food deliveries; therefore a 7-day supply of foodstuffs was stocked.

Unexpected problems were encountered with all of these three vital areas. In retrospect this is not surprising since the fury of this storm had not been equaled in the last hundred years. First, when the storm abated, the water supply system was inoperative not only for the hospital but for the entire community. Provision of water became a matter of daily poststorm planning. The entire electrical grid system for the coastal area was rendered inoperative, and the only electrical supply was by generator. The capacity of the generator and the wiring of emergency circuits was such that no power was available for elevator operation; also the air conditioning and ventilation system for the three-story building (without operable windows) was completely inoperative. Patient and staff comfort and health became a real concern as temperatures rose. Serious problems were averted by emergency procurement of individual electric fans for patient rooms and common areas, but conditions were still uncomfortable. Soup and sandwiches became the order of the day, as the contents of unpowered freezers were consumed or thrown away due to spoilage.

These problems made it essential that the hospital executive team (physician, nurse, and administrator) communicated frequently as planning was necessary to solve the problems of a changing environment.

Safety Concerns During the Hurricane

When the wind speeds surpassed gale force and approached hurricane velocity around the facility, it became apparent that windows might be broken or blown out, and flooding became a certainty. Because the winds reached velocities between 100 and 130 mph and were hurling large debris about, many outer widows were cracked, causing fear and anxiety for both patients and staff. Staff members were encouraged to spend as much time as possible on the units with the patients, attempting to attend to both medical and psychiatric needs as well as helping with concerns about the fate of loved ones or friends who were experiencing the hurricane elsewhere. At the height of the storm a staff member was assigned to each patient room. A physician the patients knew made frequent rounds as well.

At the height of the storm patients and staff became increasingly anxious about the windows in the patient rooms and considered moving the patients to an inner hallway. The hospital administrator, who was familiar with the design of the hospital, met with the patients and staff and provided calm, clear, and concise information on the design and safety of the building. This communication, offered in the middle of the night during the peak danger, served to relieve anxiety, and the patients returned to their rooms, some to sleep through the night.

Nursing

The role of nursing management before, during, and after the storm was to support, facilitate, and care for the caretakers and facilitate their professional activities (Stuart and Huggins 1990). In the face of enormous personal anxiety, grief, and loss, the providers of patient care were obligated to continue to provide care. For example, some staff members suffered total loss of their homes, and others suffered extensive damage. The executive committee decided early in the planning process that its best role was to be available for consultation and to monitor problem solving, leaving the clinical decisions in the hands of the clinicians. We elected to work in shifts with someone available around the clock. Again, planning, communications, and flexibility were paramount.

Since the medical center disaster plan designated all nursing staff as essential, we began preparations with a full complement of staff.

Child care was an immediate issue. Many of our nurses were single parents with sole responsibility for their children. Although we recommended that children be left with relatives or another parent when possible, we decided to allow those who had no alternative to bring children to the institute. A plan was developed to house the children within the second-floor youth division when the parent was not available. The staff on that unit assumed responsibility for the staff children. This became an area in which nursing management was called on to "roll up their sleeves" and help when necessary. When the manager entered the unit as helper she became subject to the direction of the nurse in charge of the unit.

As staff members began arriving armed with overnight bags, pillows, and blankets, another problem arose. Where were they to be housed? Based on the observation of a nurse manager that people respond better to crisis if they have personal space to call their own, we elected to allow staff to fan out in the institute and to find a place to "nest." We found that groups of people would congregate together in various rooms and claim territory. This seemed to be a critical factor that allowed staff to find some comfort in the face of disaster.

After the storm we recommended that the staff who were left homeless by the storm should move into the empty first-floor unit. Some, however, were reluctant to leave the nests they had built elsewhere. We continued to offer shelter for staff to stay for a week after the storm.

On the recommendation from nursing, the executive team made the decision not to accept new admissions for several days in order to provide time to nurture and support the nursing staff.

Psychologists and social workers volunteered to meet with interested staff daily to assist them with their own issues of recovery. These groups continued for about 2 weeks after the hurricane.

Medicine

Twenty-four hours before landfall of Hurricane Hugo, we recruited one psychiatrist from the attending staff for each of the three clinical units to be in charge of the medical care of the remaining patients who could not be evacuated. Thus each physician had responsibility for a defined patient population. The census of 80% occupancy 3 days before the hurricane was decreased by evacuation to 40% by the time of final

preparations for the hurricane's arrival. Because of our physical separation from the main hospital, we also recruited a physician trained in
basic life support and advanced cardiac support to prepare for the
possibility of medical emergencies.

In addition, we arranged with the hospital pharmacy to provide a
1-week supply of medication for all patients remaining during the
disaster. A pharmacy worker remained at the hospital and operated the
pharmacy efficiently throughout the disaster. All Mayday carts and
equipment were double-checked to ensure sufficient medical materials
for treatment of medical complications of psychiatric illness, such as
dehydration and infection.

The psychiatric staff also considered the possibility of the need to
treat our own staff members for any anxiety and agitation that might
occur, but did not make formal arrangements for this. This was an
important issue to consider because the impact of the hurricane on
patients and staff was greater than anticipated. The possible treatment
needs of staff should be an area of consideration for future disaster
planning.

Aftermath

After the storm, we assessed the physical damage to the building and
the physical or mental problems of the patients and staff. By now the
twice-daily meetings of the executive committee had evolved a format
that included the following agenda items:

- Clinical review (patient problems and issues)
- Staff review (general problems and issues, expanded to include
  identification of those individuals who needed housing, clothing,
  and so on)
- Task assessment (identifying jobs needing to be done)
- Task assignment
- Rumor control

Another communication tool was a daily meeting with all staff. We
began to hold this meeting the day after the storm to keep staff informed
about our situation and to answer their questions. This was an extremely useful undertaking, and we recommend that such meetings
begin immediately after a disaster such as Hugo.

Process

In retrospect, the administrative structure of our facility was critical to the success of managing the problems of a natural disaster. The twice-daily meetings held before and after the hurricane allowed dissemination of information, providing a systemic rather than discipline-specific analysis of the situation and facilitating discipline-integrated problem solving. The collaborative nature of the leadership minimized any tendency to blame others when anxious. The energy of the entire staff was directed toward constructive problem solving and caring for patients rather than venting anger and frustration.

The following vignette relates the experience of one of our nurse managers (M. Spencer, personal communication, October 1990) who remained at the institute during Hugo.

Some folks may find it difficult to associate positive feelings with a natural disaster, but working in a psychiatric facility in the midst of a hurricane (the likes of which had not been experienced in 100 years) provided some grist for the fond memories mill. Designated essential personnel had been notified to report to work and prepare to stay for the duration. As staff arrived to work at 6:30 A.M. on the morning of September 21, laden with sleeping bags, peanut butter, and bags of chocolate chip cookies, I was struck by the panorama of their responses to our surreal situation. Comments ranged from "Boy is this gonna be fun" to "Ain't no way I'm staying here." Several staff who were too anxious to work were sent home. Ironically, several patients who could have elected to go home decided to stay at the institute, feeling safer in the hospital. The last place I wanted to be was on the Charleston peninsula, riding out a category 4 hurricane during high tide, but such was my lot in life at the time. My husband and I had just moved into our first home earlier in the week, conveniently located in the flood zone. I now was obligated to leave spouse and cat behind to stay with my mother while I reported for work. As I concluded that I probably wouldn't have a house left, I set about to do my job and cursed the rotten timing of my home ownership.

The morning of the hurricane was spent preparing for the siege that lay ahead. The patients from the first floor were moved to the third floor due to the possibility of flooding. The attending physician with whom I worked on a daily basis decided to do chart rounds and walk round as usual to provide some sense of structure and to continue to care for the patients. Our interdisciplinary team of sometimes a dozen players was whittled down to the two of us. It was business as usual, if only for an hour or so.

The evening brought a sense of tension, apprehension, and anticipation, as we all wondered where the storm would land. Several of us gathered in a classroom to watch television, just to relax and get some diversion. Scanning the tube, I decided to watch baseball: The Chicago Cubs in Wrigley Field. Somehow, it was comforting to know that someone, somewhere in the world was having fun at a ball game, while we wondered what would happen to us over the next several hours. Around the seventh-inning stretch, another viewer insisted on watching the Weather Channel to track the gargantuan storm in the Atlantic. I knew we were sitting ducks; I didn't need the weather report to remind me, and I really preferred baseball. Someone decided to post a sign-up list for television times. I decided to go to bed around 10 P.M. or so, feeling that I needed to be fresh in the morning, not up to fighting over what to watch, and believing erroneously that I could sleep during the whole thing.

Another nurse and myself had set up camp in a social worker's office on the third floor, the top floor of the institute. As I got ready for bed, I thought "Why me? How did I get myself into this? This is the last time I go into a helping profession." By this time, the wind and rain intensified. As I stretched out, well away from the windows, watching the sky illuminating from lightening and exploding transformers, I thought I detected the gentle movement of the floor beneath me. "Nonsense," I muttered. Abruptly, the floor began to vibrate, the walls started to breathe, and the entire building commenced to rumble like a freight train. I flew out of the room along with the rest of the nurses in the adjacent offices—afraid that otherwise I'd get sucked out the window.

The attending physician was in the charting room, feet propped up, calmly documenting. The building continued to rumble, and a rhythmic pounding on the roof was deafening. The physician commented that buildings were constructed to sway and that the sound on the roof was gravel being buffeted by the wind. I was skeptical. The medical director explained that the vents on the roof were clattering back and forth. I was not convinced. It felt as if the building would collapse. Around this time, the staff had moved the patients off the unit and into the third-floor waiting area. There was a fear that the windows in their rooms would blow out, but the fears were unfounded. Standing in the middle of the patients and staff was the hospital administrator—a down-to-earth, gray-bearded gent from Tennessee with a lovely southern accent who took great pride in the structural integrity of the building. Prior to the opening of the institute in 1988, he would take interested parties on guided tours of the incomplete hospital, calling one's attention to the intricate electrical system or the finely crafted plumbing. Now, there he stood, giving a midnight soliloquy in the eerie darkness of the waiting room, highlighting the institute's safety features—particularly the unbreakable windows that were "several sheets thick." Patients and staff listened attentively; there was an aura of ghost stories around the campfire. He was as reassuring as the baseball game had been earlier in the evening. Patients and staff returned to their rooms. When the eye of the storm passed over us, we couldn't resist venturing outside for a peek. The water was rushing down the street like a river, well up to the top of the parking meters. Debris, stingray, and assorted fish were spotted; someone commented on a range and refrigerator. Everyone started to laugh at the ridiculous situation.

Around 2 A.M., after the storm had passed, I lay down only to be awakened at 5:30 A.M. to no electricity, no water, and no air conditioning. The emergency generator had not yet kicked in, but did so eventually—still leaving us without air conditioning. The staff received instructions on flushing the commodes after every fifth use only. Our clinical nurse manager and director of nursing later volunteered to scoop out the toilets when the situation warranted—the former wearing shorts and running shoes, the latter in a dress in sneakers—both of them sporting stained latex gloves.

Conclusions

The leadership in this disaster was concerned first with the care of the patients, second with the care of the caretakers, and third with the smooth operation of the system as a whole. When disaster occurred, the focus on communication, planning, and flexibility worked well for the existing management structure. We recommend that hospitals provide constant communications between medicine, nursing, and hospital administration during a disaster. If a structure for such communication does not already exist, frequent regularly scheduled meetings help not only with information transfer but with group problem solving and support.

Reference

Stuart G, Huggins E: Caring for the caretakers in times of disaster. Journal of Child and Adolescent Psychiatric Nursing 3:144–147, 1990

Additional Readings

Laube J, Murphy S: Perspectives on Disaster Recovery. Norwalk, CT, Appleton-Century Crofts, 1985

Lystad, M: Mental Health Response to Mass Emergencies. New York, Brunner/Mazel, 1989

Sowder B, Lystad M: Disaster and Mental Health. Washington, DC, American Psychiatric Press, 1985

Wright K, Ursano R, Bartone P, et al: The shared experience of catastrophe: an expanded classification of the disaster community. Am J Orthopsychiatry 60:35–42, 1990

Chapter 13

Tornado in Eastern North Carolina: Outreach to School and Community

Lesly Tamarin Mega, M.D.
Susan Lynn McCammon, Ph.D.

*O*n March 28, 1984, tornadoes ripped through North Carolina and South Carolina; 44 people were killed, 800 were injured, and 2,200 were left temporarily without homes. One of the tornadoes touched down in eastern North Carolina at about 9:25 P.M. for 22 miles, cutting a path one-fourth to one-half mile wide. As a result, 9 people died, and 153 were injured; property damage was estimated in the millions in Pitt County. The area was taken by surprise by the disaster as tornadoes were virtually unheard of there, and warnings were rare and ineffectual.

Pitt County has a population of less than 50,000. Although it is rural, it has a regional state university with approximately 16,000 students and a medical school with 60–80 students per class. It is the site of a tertiary hospital with a well-established emergency medicine department and a comprehensive mental health center.

Because the disaster was a sudden, unpredicted, and unusual occurrence, the community was unprepared physically and emotionally to cope with the enormity of its impact. The existing disaster plans were geared toward functioning at the scene of a disaster; however, the

We appreciate the participation of Sudhakar Madakasira, M.D.—Psychiatry Research Consultant; David Ames, M.D., Steven Creech, Ph.D., and Randy Horton, M.S.—Pitt County Mental Health Center Administrators; and Leslie Parker, M.S., Sylvia Mullis, M.D., Beth Vail, M.S., Marsha Mills, B.A., and Laura Ferguson—Project FOCUS Staff. Project FOCUS was supported by NIMH Grant 1 HO7 MH000016-01.

victims were scattered over a 10- to 12-mile radius (Williamson and Allison 1984). Emergency rescue service was hampered because of the dark, windy, rainy weather conditions; the presence of fallen trees and debris; and the lack of telephone service. The hospital's emergency department became the primary scene of disaster interventions. As a result of the tornado, some workplaces had limited access, and some schools needing repairs were closed. The population was stunned and confused by the disaster.

Initial Response

Despite lack of preparation, the community and professional response was dramatically effective and supportive. Temporary shelter and donated food and clothing were immediately offered. On the night of the tornado, 500 of the victims' friends and relatives waiting in the medical center hospital cafeteria were helped by members of the hospital's social service and administration departments (Williamson and Allison 1984). At the same time, the mental health center set up a crisis intervention team in the auditorium close to the emergency department. The team provided information and support for families and victims with minor injuries and encouraged the families to share experiences (Madakasira et al. 1985).

The day after the tornado the mental health center began to plan follow-up interventions, with consultation from East Carolina University's (ECU) psychiatrists and psychologists and from a Duke University graduate psychology student with expertise in disaster assistance programs. Discussions about potential emotional reactions to the tornado were planned and conducted with area leaders, such as the mayor and clergy, and with caregivers, including members of the departments of social services and public health, the Red Cross, fire and rescue squads, nurses, and physicians. Pamphlets describing possible stress reactions to the trauma were given to these groups to be distributed in the community.

Mental health center personnel stationed themselves at the disaster assistance centers set up by the federal government to educate victims departing from the centers on mental health treatment resources in the community. As reported at other disasters, the mental health center staff discovered secondary traumatization of victims because of the complications involved in the process of obtaining governmental remuneration. To help victims express their feelings and discuss their experiences with others, the mental health center staff set up group sessions at various public schools in the area (Madakasira et al. 1985).

The media and the telephone were other important sources of education and support to the community. Headlines included "Here's How You Can Aid Victims of Tornadoes" (1984) and "ECU Offers Free Psychiatric Care to Tornado Victims" (Hendrick 1984). Toll-free numbers were advertised to donate money or goods, such as food, furniture, appliances, and household supplies; and addresses were given for a newly established North Carolina Tornado Victim Housing Fund and Disaster Relief Funds. Professionals spoke on television and radio about possible stress reactions and symptoms to expect, and television meteorologists explained tornado weather patterns and plans for taking proper precautions in the event of future tornadoes. A national television broadcast was aired after a reporter interviewed parents, teachers, and schoolchildren about their reactions to the tornado. The Real Crisis Center, a regular telephone crisis service sponsored by the United Way, increased its volunteer services by offering a tornado-related telephone hot line.

Follow-Up Services: Outreach Model

The major emphasis of the early crisis intervention period was to provide psychological first aid (Frederick 1977; Slaikeu 1984). Although the mental health center and the ECU Department of Psychiatric Medicine offered free services, relatively few people responded; only about 40 people attended the various school-based educational and support sessions. Because of this and the reports of others that people are reluctant to use mental health services after disasters (Lindy et al. 1981), school and community outreach programs were developed to provide intervention for more people.

The Pitt County intervention program was developed according to crisis theory and other models of secondary prevention as described by Caplan (1964). The goals of our outreach programs were to decrease both immediate and delayed stress reactions and symptoms by encouraging expression of thoughts and feelings about the trauma, offering social support and a sense of connection to the community, and supplying techniques to allow emotional mastery of the traumatic events. Because we were cognizant that roles, tasks, and agencies would change throughout the stages of disaster recovery (Hartsough 1982), assessments of needs were made the salient focus of the outreach efforts. The desire to reach more people in this small community was motivated by the observation that everyone was affected in one way or another by the impact of the tornado and by the natural disaster literature, which described the necessity for crisis interventions to decrease stress and enhance coping mechanisms.

Specific components of our outreach project were gleaned from previous projects designed to respond to natural and human-made disasters. These included the following: Project Outreach following the 1972 Hurricane Agnes flood in Pennsylvania (Heffron 1977; Okura 1975; Richard 1974), the Monticello Neighbor-to-Neighbor Team developed in response to Indiana tornadoes (Zarle et al. 1974), and the mental health response to the Hyatt Regency skywalk collapse in Kansas City in 1981 (Gist and Stolz 1982; Wilkinson 1983). We also made liberal use of National Institute of Mental Health (NIMH) disaster services publications (Farberow and Frederick 1983; Farberow and Gordon 1981; National Institute of Mental Health 1984; Tierney and Baisden 1983).

Follow-Up Services: Children's School Outreach Project—Teachers as "Therapists"

Initiation of School Outreach

The Children's School Outreach Project was created by ECU psychiatrists and Pitt County Mental Health Center professionals. The use of school personnel to detect symptoms and to provide support and education for our community's children seemed to be the natural route to take to reach as many children as possible. We were encouraged in this by requests from several schools asking for guidance for their faculty and staff on how to help their children cope with the posttraumatic effects of the tornado. Their descriptions included "a kindergartner who hides in a cubbyhole afraid to come out," "a 6-year-old who screams incessantly when she hears thunder to drown out her fear of the storm," "a first grader who suddenly refuses to leave his mother to go to school," and "a teenager who balances books on his head to protect himself from falling objects."

A meeting was quickly arranged with the county's superintendent of schools and other school officials to explain and get approval for our intervention program. Less than 2 weeks after the tornado, a team of psychiatrists and mental health center professionals conducted seminars with faculty and staff from seven county schools. Four of the schools were in the area directly hit by the tornado; three were in areas close by. The schools included elementary and middle schools, with children from ages 5 to 16 in grades kindergarten to eighth grade. In some of the schools the guidance counselors requested to meet with us before we met with the group.

Training Workshop

The school principals, counselors, and teachers were told that we were meeting with them to help them learn to identify the children's emotional reactions to the tornado and how they could help the children. It was explained that they were in the best position of anyone to help the community's children, for they were with them each day in their natural setting and could detect changes in their behavior. They were told that they were also victims of the tornado and that it was necessary for them to recognize their emotional reactions and symptoms in order to help the children effectively. We encouraged them to meet on a regular basis to support each other and to consult with us if they felt the need.

We described symptoms of posttraumatic stress disorder. Immediately after, a principal of one of the schools shared that since the tornado he experienced "a tightening in his stomach whenever bad rains were predicted." A teacher then spoke of dreaming about "being sucked into the toilet"; during the tornado, she witnessed the water in the toilet being sucked out by its force. Sharing of experiences such as these was encouraged.

The group was informed that children vary in their susceptibility and reactions to traumatic events: "A child who lost his home may have a less obvious immediate reaction than the child who knew someone who lost everything but didn't suffer material damage himself; however, the first child might have a significant delayed reaction." Further, they were told that the children most at risk for emotional reactions were those children who lost family members, friends, or pets; those who were physically injured; those who felt they were in extreme danger; those who had experienced previous disasters; or those who had personal or family-related emotional problems before the tornado. It was explained: "During a disaster, parents or adult volunteers might have been so preoccupied by responsibilities for obtaining food, clothing, shelter, and safety that they could have been unaware of or unable to fulfill the child's needs for love, information, understanding, or a sense of belonging. If this occurred, symptoms could be more likely to occur."

Questionnaires as Educational, Therapeutic, and Research Tools

The school personnel were informed that two questionnaires had been specifically formulated for the children and parents (by L. T. Mega and S. Madakasira). It was explained:

> These questionnaires will serve the purpose of educating you, the children, and the parents about what symptoms to expect. They can be the springboard for a discussion with your students and for the parents for discussion with their children. They can help you identify students with symptoms so that they can get appropriate help. Of course your direct observations of a nervous child or a child whose behavior has changed in any way, for instance, from outgoing to quiet or vice versa, are more important. The questionnaire will also serve as a research tool to help us determine if the children are actually upset and if we are looking for the right symptoms.

The questionnaires for both the children and parents consisted of questions written in children's language paralleling DSM-III (American Psychiatric Association 1980) criteria for posttraumatic stress disorder. Some DSM-III criteria were not used because they were too difficult to express in language that a child could understand or the criteria were observable rather than reportable symptoms. Added to the parents' questionnaires were three extra questions regarding their children: avoidance of reminders of the tornado, intensification of symptoms from symbolic exposure to the trauma, and previous history of emotional problems. Also included were questions about anticipation of the disaster recurring without specifying a stimulus, irritability and agitation, sadness, separation anxiety, change in appetite, and self-blame or magical thinking (i.e., children might have thought that the tornado occurred because of their bad behavior).

After the children's questionnaire was distributed and reviewed with the school personnel, a teacher's instruction page for administering it was circulated. It instructed the teachers to explain that the questionnaire is not a test, that its purpose is to find out how the tornado has affected the children so that we can help them, that it is about their feelings since the tornado, and that it should be answered honestly. The teacher was asked to read each question aloud to the class, to start with the sample questions, and to allow the students enough time to fill in the appropriate spaces.

A parents' questionnaire was similarly distributed. It was explained that the questionnaire would serve the same purpose for the parents as the children's questionnaire served for the teachers. It could also help identify those children with symptoms who could not answer their questionnaire for whatever reason (e.g., not understanding, afraid to admit to problems), could open the door for communication between the parents and the school, and could allow us to correlate the parents' perceptions of their children's symptoms with their children's perceptions.

At the end of the parent questionnaire was space for the parents to describe their reaction to the tornado. This was included because of the assumption that often a child's reaction reflects the way his or her parents are coping. With this information, we hoped to understand better the particular child's reactions. We also hoped that this would inform the parents that it was appropriate for them to have reactions to the tornado and that we could offer assistance if they experienced symptoms. During the 2–6 weeks after the tornado, 3,752 children and 2,284 parents were surveyed.

Other Classroom Strategies

Following the discussion of the questionnaires with the school personnel, a handout prepared in Santa Cruz County, California, describing children's symptoms and treatment options in the various age groups (National Institute of Mental Health 1984) was distributed and briefly explained. It was emphasized that children's interpretation of their environment is dependent on their age and experience and it is most important to allow for expression of thoughts and feelings. This led to the discussion of concrete ways to help the children in the classroom besides the use of the questionnaire.

Three basic guidelines were followed: to allow expression of thoughts and feelings, to supply support and a sense of social connection, and to utilize techniques for psychic mastery. It was believed that this approach could help the children gain control over their feelings of total helplessness.

To illustrate how the teachers could help the children in their classrooms, one teacher's experience was described. All of us were familiar with this teacher's reaction to the tornado because it was aired on national television. Aware that Ms. L. had also shared her personal experience with her class, I related this to the other school personnel (with her permission). She described, "I became panicky every time it was ready to storm or when a storm was forecasted. During the tornado the windows shook, pictures fell off the wall, and when I ran to take cover in the bathroom, I could have sworn that the tornado was in there with me." A newspaper article describing the tornado, weather charts, and tornado drill information hung from her classroom wall. Her disclosure served to provide the children with an open and honest communication from a caring adult and demonstrated that it was permissible to have a reaction to this terrible event. Ms. L.'s discussion of the tornado with her class each day, as more news became available, continued to allow for feelings to be expressed. It also kept the students informed, providing a sense of inclusion and social connection, and supplied information that helped them better understand. For those children who did not feel comfortable speaking up in class, Ms. L. encouraged them to express their feelings through writing a composition on the tornado.

The teachers were taught additional ways to encourage their students to express their feelings. We adapted for use in our school system both a list of classroom activities used by teachers in California Bay area counties after a disastrous storm in January 1982 (National Institute of Mental Health 1984) and Crabbs's (1981) classroom intervention strategies. One suggestion was to ask the children to finish sentences such as: "During the tornado, I was scared when _____; When I lost my _____, I felt _____; or When it rains, I think about _____" (Crabbs 1981). The teachers could follow this activity with a discussion about what was written.

Other approaches included asking the children to draw pictures of things that remind them of a tornado, to draw as a group a mural entitled "The Tornado of 1984" on large pieces of butcher paper, and to make a "magic" box from a covered shoe box to pass around asking the children to wish for various things, such as to locate their most important lost item in the tornado (Crabbs 1981) or to change a feeling they might be experiencing. For kindergartners and first graders, play activities were described as more effective and less frightening than discussions. A tornado game could be created in which the children or puppets could act as a tornado, the people, the buildings, or the helpers.

Reassurance and preparation help the mastery process. Reassuring the children that the tornado is not a regular occurrence was important. It was explained that the teachers might say, "We don't expect it to happen again, but if it ever does, let's prepare for it." Inviting a fire fighter, rescue squad worker, or weather forecaster to class to discuss either how to predict a tornado or how to prepare for one was suggested. To decrease guilt and enhance support and social connection, the teachers could plan with the children ways to help those who suffered loss by making or donating a toy or donating clothing.

It was stressed that there were some positive aspects of the disaster. The children were made aware of the community support and effort and of the emotional support available. School personnel were told that we speculate that the traumas from this disaster will be less severe because of the pulling together of people in the area.

Besides looking for current symptoms, the school personnel were encouraged to continue to watch for delayed reactions. It was explained that some children would appear to be okay now, but that subsequently their grades could drop or their behavior could change in other ways. Recommendations were made to continue to keep the normal school routine, but to be flexible. "Take time to talk about the feelings and facts concerning the tornado and don't expect perfection from the children. Some will not be able to do their best." Because statewide achievement tests were scheduled during this time, the school personnel were warned that the trauma from the tornado might influence the scores and that this might have to be taken into consideration if these scores were used for class placement.

The discussion ended with plans to administer the questionnaires to the children, to distribute the parent questionnaires, and to try some versions of the various discussion techniques proposed. School personnel were encouraged to refer the more troubled children, parents, or families to guidance counselors or to the ECU child psychiatrist or the children's division of the mental health center.

Follow-Up Sessions

The training workshops resulted in follow-up meetings with some of the school counselors, teachers, and the ECU child psychiatrist for suggestions on how to handle individual children. Some children and parents were referred for treatment.

> Paul J., a 6-and-a-half-year-old who lived with his mother, father, and sister, was seen 5 weeks after the tornado struck near his home. One week after the tornado his mother described him as "overanxious and easily frightened, concerned about another tornado striking and becoming separated from us." He didn't want to leave his mother to go to school and had refused to ride the school bus. Normally an excellent student, he was reading less at home, his reading grade dropped, and he was not thoroughly completing his assignments. He turned off news programs concerning the tornado and avoided talking about it.
>
> Paul's mother, a nurse, was called into work on the night of the tornado to help families identify tornado victims. When she thought about the tornado she became very upset and often cried. She was helped by talking about her feelings with her husband. Notably, the family history was significant for suicides among second-degree relatives.
>
> When first seen, Paul was shy, timid, and whiny. When his mother was talking to the therapist, he frequently interrupted and wanted to leave. Alone with the therapist, he explained that talking about the tornado scared him and admitted that he was having some difficulties as a result. However, he explained that he wasn't going to school because other students were picking on him, even though there was no evidence of this. He was subdued and anxious, and his picture drawing showed signs of overcontrol. The parents' questionnaire indicated positive symptoms and signs.
>
> Paul J. was seen four times after the initial interview. He was at first reluctant to separate from his mother. His play was not spontaneous, and he avoided reference to the tornado. On his second visit, he began to separate more easily and was confident that he was upset about his parents wanting him to play baseball rather than about the tornado. On the third visit, he described fighting back at school and others being scared of him. He said, "I'm not worried about the tornado because I come here and I'm cured." On the last visit both he and his mother agreed that he had improved, but under certain circumstances, such as watching the *Wizard of Oz*, he develops a "stomachache." It was agreed that he would return as needed.

Project Evaluation

A teacher's survey was developed by Drs. Mega and Madakasira to evaluate this school intervention program. Of the 61 teachers who responded, 93% reported valuable discussions resulting from this approach. More than 50% of the teachers reported spending up to 3 hours in classroom discussion on activities regarding the disaster.

Tornado Follow-Up and Community Support: Project FOCUS

Initiation of Community Outreach

A month after the tornado, the North Carolina Department of Mental Health, Mental Retardation and Substance Abuse Services convened a meeting of representatives from community mental health centers in catchment areas affected by the tornadoes. Information was disseminated regarding potential funding and proposal guidelines for a crisis counseling grant awarded and administered by NIMH and funded by the Federal Emergency Management Administration (FEMA). The mental health department submitted a proposal describing the development of an outreach staff to seek out tornado survivors and to conduct an assessment of mental health and material needs. The outreach workers were then to facilitate linkage with appropriate community and federal resources. We eagerly awaited the speedy funding that was promised, but the official award was not made until July, 4 months after the tornadoes. (We understand the turnaround time is much quicker now, and emergency funding is more immediately available.)

The staffing plan was revised due to the delay, and the staff members were recruited and hired. In early August, 2 days of training were organized by Bonnie Morell, M.S.W., M.R.P. (of the Department of Mental Health), for the Eastern North Carolina region. This training session was attended by community mental health center project staff, state officials, and representatives from NIMH and FEMA. Wayne Richard, Ph.D., Coordinator of Mental Health Disaster Preparedness, Tennessee Department of Mental Health and Mental Retardation, presented an overview on mental health follow-up to disasters.

The Pitt County Mental Health Center project was named *Tornado Followup and Community Support* (Project FOCUS). The staff participated in further orientation and training. The staff consisted of a project coordinator (full-time, 6 months), a field coordinator (full-time, 4 months), two outreach workers (full-time, 3 months), and a part-time secretary. All four of the full-time workers conducted the outreach visits. They were supervised by a part-time psychologist consultant (4 hours per week) and the director of community services. Two psychiatrists also served as consultants, one primarily regarding needs assessment and symptom measures and the other regarding issues and selected cases involving children.

Preparation for Fieldwork

Project staff initiated contact with relevant agencies to determine available resources (e.g., FEMA/Temporary Housing Authority, Salvation Army, Community Action, hospital county disaster offices, ministerial association). A listing of those affected by the tornado was obtained from the disaster assistance centers, the tax supervisor's office, and referral from other agencies and community members. A structured interview format was developed and pretested to assess tornado impact, level and sources of social support, and unmet needs of tornado survivors. Information was gathered and a FOCUS pamphlet was printed, which was distributed to all households visited. Included in the pamphlet were sections on common reactions to disaster (Kansas City Association for Mental Health 1983), suggestions for handling fear of storms (McCammon 1984), information for parents to help their children (developed by Corder and Haizlip 1984), tornado safety tips (National Oceanic and Atmospheric Administration 1979), and information on relaxation and meditation (various sources). A coloring book called "After the Tornado" (Corder and Haizlip 1984) was distributed to families with children from 2 to 7 years old, along with a book list of stories about disaster and survival for elementary, junior, and senior high levels. In addition, adults in the household received a letter inviting them to complete two questionnaires—Hopkins's brief self-report symptom inventory (Derogatis et al. 1974) and Horowitz and Wilner's Coping Inventory (1981)—and return them in stamped envelopes. Finally, a summary form was developed to record what transpired during each contact with the family.

Publicizing the project was another part of preparation for fieldwork. Local newspapers, radio, and television were used to inform the community members about Project FOCUS and to alert them to expect the visits from outreach workers. A letter of endorsement from local and district government officials and ministers was published in the newspaper.

Outreach Visits

Outreach visits were initiated in September. The workers were easily admitted into the survivors' homes (or "temporary" housing) and found that people used them to listen to their experiences and to assist their emotional recovery. Even though this was months after the tornadoes, the survivors never tired of telling their stories. Many still grieved and struggled to work through powerful emotions.

Weekly staff meetings with the psychologist consultant included not only administrative concerns, but also issues of staff needs and feelings that were aroused by the often emotionally charged interviews. In addition to providing empathic listening, the staff worked with 80 of the participating 249 families to help with requests for furniture, winter clothing, fuel and housing, and counseling referral.

The following case study was included in the final report for the project (Parker 1985, p. 15).

> Mr. and Mrs. W. were both at the Portertown Church (only a mile away from their trailer) the night of the tornado. They lost everything except the clothes on their backs. This was extremely difficult for the W.'s because Mr. W. was over 60, and Mrs. W. couldn't work because of severe arthritis. More than anything, they wanted to leave their FEMA trailer and return to their own lot.
>
> At the time of their initial interview, the obvious unmet needs were obtaining permanent housing, replacing household items and clothing they had lost. Not quite as apparent were the emotional needs. Mrs. W. had severe storm anxieties and had been on "nerve" medication ever since her mother's death several years prior. She agreed to attend a support group to learn how to combat these fears and followed through with that promise and is improving her coping skills.
>
> As far as the more material needs, the Lion's Club International awarded money to purchase clothing; the Disaster Relief Fund donated monies to help replace household furnishing and appliances; FEMA—Temporary Housing is pleading their case before the Unmet Needs Committee to help obtain permanent housing; Mrs. W. has turned to Project FOCUS on numerous occasions just to talk, for

empathy, and direction. Mr. and Mrs. W. finally received a check for $4,000.00 from IFG (Individual Family Grant), giving them a down payment for a new trailer.

Support Groups

Of the 63 home visits completed by the third week in September (6 months posttornado), three-fourths of the respondents indicated an interest in support groups. Planning was initiated for three groups, organized by geographic areas. Meetings were held in a school library, a church education building, and a fire station. Leaders were recruited, and additional funding was requested. Facilitators were local mental health professionals, and a nonprofessional cofacilitator from the affected area was identified for each group based on the recommendations of outreach project staff. Orientation and periodic meetings were held for facilitators. The support groups began October 30 and held weekly meetings until the Christmas season. Then they met again on the 1-year anniversary of the tornadoes.

The initial meeting of each group was begun by a brief presentation on common reactions to disaster. Handouts were distributed, and the participants were encouraged to discuss whether their own reactions were similar to any listed by the facilitator. Group participants quickly began to join in through telling their stories or listening intently. The emphasis was on providing a forum for sharing experiences and feelings, with the opportunity to tell one's story. A fellowship atmosphere was cultivated, and eventually most groups began to meet in homes of members. Educational interventions included providing information on weather, tornado safety, available resources for material and financial assistance, and stages of grief. A problem-solving stance was taught, including help with problem identification, setting priorities, brainstorming, and identifying steps to carry out a solution. Members often reported accomplishments since the previous meeting. Separate activities were held for the children while the adults met. Children's activities included use of the tornado coloring books, bibliotherapy (using books with themes of children coping with difficult situations), art projects, and games.

Outreach project staff provided support services by handling administrative tasks, obtaining materials and refreshments, publicizing meetings, providing transportation, and attending group meetings. The psychology consultant attended some meetings to provide supervision and to support facilitators. In addition, she facilitated the meetings of the group leaders, who convened monthly to discuss the progress of the groups, share strategies and problems, and support each other.

Although originally planned to last just 6 weeks, additional meetings were held by two of the groups. Although attendance fluctuated (ranging at sessions from 2 to 25 participants), the groups had a faithful core of participants who continued to be involved throughout the series. Initial meetings brought the highest attendance; for some people, coming to one meeting apparently satisfied their need to learn that their reactions and problems were not atypical. Over time the focus of the groups shifted toward meeting social and fellowship needs rather than narrow attention to the tornado, although the tornado continued to be the unifying theme.

Project Outcome and Evaluation

Project staff reported serving 249 families with counseling and education. Nearly $15,000 in small grants of financial assistance was issued by the Disaster Relief Fund and Lions Club to meet needs identified by project staff. Fifty-six people participated in either the support groups or in individual therapy at the mental health center. Even though the support groups were initiated late after the disaster (7 months posttornado), they still seemed to meet important needs and address issues yet unresolved. A postgroup evaluation revealed several aspects to be most helpful, including talking about the storm and weather, relieving some of the fear and pressure by talking, and securing needed financial and medical help. One participant wrote on his evaluation, "It has been a real experience for me in that I believe this group saved my life, and I'll be forever grateful." Another said that the five meetings he attended were very helpful to him because he was "a nervous wreck."

A subsequent analysis of the symptom data (reported by Madakasira and O'Brien 1987) revealed endorsement of symptom patterns consistent with criteria for posttraumatic stress disorder in 63% of those who returned the symptom checklists at approximately 5 months posttornado. Although a more prompt intervention would have been preferable, it was clear that substantial needs still existed and that at least some people were still amenable to help.

Follow-Up Studies

In a research study separate from the outreach component, 120 rescue and hospital personnel responded to a survey of their emotional reactions and coping behaviors subsequent to the tornado. Workers reported many of the symptoms of posttraumatic stress disorder, most frequently reporting repetitive intrusive thoughts. Workers at the tornado scene reported fewer symptoms than those workers at the hospital. Symptom constellations consistent with diagnostic criteria for posttraumatic stress disorder were reported by 17% of the respondents. The results of the study clearly indicated a need for support services for hospital and rescue workers involved in disaster relief (McCammon et al. 1988).

In addition, follow-up studies to the outreach components were undertaken a year after the initial questionnaires were received. Analyses and reporting on those data are in progress.

Conclusion

Although the outcome of these psychoeducational outreach programs could not be determined, the teachers and adult support group participants reported that they were helpful. The following summarizes the unique components of these programs:

- The grant provided a salaried person able to give full attention to coordinating the program. It provided the staff to conduct the needs assessment for individual families.
- The outreach staff played a unique role as the vital link between the human services agencies and the survivors. State, civic, and religious organizations had resources but were without the personnel or mechanisms to match these resources with those who needed them.
- The involvement of psychologists and psychiatrists provided the outreach staff and school personnel with programmatic and case consultation, as well as help in coping with their personal reactions and anxieties stimulated from working with victims.
- There was only one school system involved, and easy access to the schools was obtained because of the long-standing relationship of the university's child psychiatrist and the mental health center staff with the schools.

- The requests by the school and community for psychological interventions made it easier to implement the programs.
- The program offered service and provided research opportunities.
- The use of the concrete structured interventional tools (i.e., the questionnaires and structured interview format) aided in engaging, educating, and guiding the teachers, outreach workers, and families.
- The teachers were used as first-line-of-defense "therapists." They could interact with the majority of children and already had a relationship with them.
- The needs generated by the survivors created the follow-up support groups and the content for group discussion. The community outreach program appeared to be helpful to its participants even though by some standards it was late in being initiated. Although some have suggested 1–3 months as the optimal time for intervention (Lindy et al. 1981), it appeared that during the first few months some victims were preoccupied with caring for themselves physically and only after some of these needs were met did they experience increased emotional stress. Later, victims became angry and depressed because they had time to think about what had happened, the barrage of attention diminished, and remuneration was slow in coming.
- In another tornado follow-up, North et al. (1989) found that psychiatric disorders and symptom rates were low in tornado survivors who were evaluated within 1 month of the disaster. Their lack of findings may be due to the survivors' protective denial. In our experience, a significant number of adults (seen at 5 months) and children (for 2–6 weeks) described symptoms of posttraumatic stress and behavioral changes. Perhaps our population may have had to cope with a greater extent of injury and loss.

As a result of our outreach involvement, we would additionally suggest the following strategies for disaster. First, provide interventions, such as critical incident stress reduction, for emergency and hospital workers who experienced posttraumatic symptoms. Media personnel also were seen to experience these symptoms and therefore should be offered intervention measures. Second, consider the development of improved techniques to alleviate such symptoms as anticipatory fears of tornado occurrence often stimulated by rain storms. Third, quick initiation of house-to-house visits may decrease symptoms and increase the strength of group support. Fourth, share ideas with other professionals attempting to deal with the emotions surrounding a disaster. (We were unaware that a group a 90-minute drive west of us was also planning and implementing a school outreach program described by McRee et al. 1986.)

We hope that the interventions, ideas, and concerns described can be useful to others in similar situations. Perhaps our programs may serve as models for intervention and investigation of stress reactions in rural vulnerable populations.

References

American Psychiatric Association: Diagnostic and Statistical Manual of Mental Disorders, 3rd Edition. Washington, DC, American Psychiatric Association, 1980

Caplan G: Principles of Preventive Psychiatry. New York, Basic Books, 1964

Corder BF, Haizlip T: After the Tornado: A Coloring Book for Children and Their Parents or Helpers. Raleigh, NC, NC Division of Mental Health, Mental Retardation, and Substance Abuse, 1984

Crabbs MA: School mental health services following an environmental disaster. J Sch Health 51:165–167, 1981

Derogatis LR, Lipman RS, Rickels K, et al: The Hopkins Symptom Checklist (HSCL): a self-report symptom inventory. Behav Sci 19:1–15, 1974

Farberow NL, Frederick CJ: Training Manual for Human Service Workers in Major Disasters. Rockville, MD, National Institute of Mental Health, 1983

Farberow L, Gordon NS: Manual for Child Health Workers in Major Disasters. Rockville, MD, National Institute of Mental Health, 1981

Frederick CJ: Current thinking about crisis or psychological intervention in United States disasters. Mass Emergencies 2:43–50, 1977

Gist R, Stolz SB: Mental health promotion and the media: community response to the Kansas City hotel disaster. Am Psychol 37:1136–1139, 1982

Hartsough DM: Planning for disaster: a new community outreach program for mental health centers. Journal of Community Psychology 10:255–264, 1982

Heffron EF: Project Outreach: crisis intervention following natural disaster. Journal of Community Psychology 5:103–110, 1977

Hendrick G: Help is available for post-tornado stress. Greenville, NC, Daily Reflector, April 5, 1984, p 10

Here's how you can aid victims of tornadoes. Raleigh News and Observer, April 6, 1984, p 8C

Horowitz MJ, Wilner N: Life events, stress and coping, in Aging in the 80s. Edited by Poon L. Washington, DC, American Psychological Association, 1981

Kansas City Association for Mental Health: Reaction to Disaster. Kansas City, MO, Kansas City Association for Mental Health, 1983

Lindy JD, Grace MC, Green BL: Survivors: outreach to a reluctant population. Am J Orthopsychiatry 51:468–478, 1981

Madakasira S, O'Brien K: Acute post-traumatic stress disorder in victims of a natural disaster. J Nerv Ment Dis 175:286–290, 1987

Madakasira S, Ames DA, Mega LT: The 1984 tornadoes: response from the mental health profession. North Carolina Journal of Mental Health 10:17–20, 1985

McCammon S: Fear of storms. Unpublished manuscript, Greenville, NC, East Carolina University, Department of Psychology, 1984

McCammon S, Durham TW, Allison EJ, et al: Emergency workers' cognitive appraisal and coping with traumatic events. Journal of Traumatic Stress 1:353–372, 1988

McRee C, Deitz S, Silverstein E, et al: A preliminary report on short term intervention with children and parents in a tornado disaster area. Psychiatric Forum 13:86–90, 1986

National Institute of Mental Health: Counseling Programs for Children Following Major Disasters. Rockville, MD, NIMH Center for Mental Health Studies of Emergencies, 1984

National Oceanic and Atmospheric Administration: Tornado safety in residences (NOAA/PA 79016). Washington, DC, U.S. Government Printing Office, 1979

North CS, Smith EM, McCool RE, et al: Acute postdisaster coping and adjustment. Journal of Traumatic Stress 2:353–360, 1989

Okura KP: Mobilizing in response to a major disaster. Community Ment Health J 11:136–144, 1975

Parker L: Project FOCUS: final report. Greenville, NC, Pitt County Mental Health, Mental Retardation and Substance Abuse Services, 1985

Richard WC: Crisis intervention services following natural disaster: the Pennsylvania recovery project. Journal of Community Psychology 2:211–219, 1974

Slaikeu KA: Crisis Intervention: A Handbook for Practice and Research. Boston, MA, Allyn & Bacon, 1984

Tierney KJ, Baisden B: Crisis intervention programs for disaster victims: a source book and manual for smaller communities. Rockville, MD, National Institute of Mental Health, 1983

Wilkinson CB: Symptomatic aftermath of a disaster: Hyatt Regency Hotel skywalk collapse. Am J Psychiatry 140:1134–1139, 1983

Williamson JE, Allison EJ Jr: Disaster plan implementation: tornadoes strike eastern North Carolina. N C Med J 45:434–436, 1984

Chapter 14

Research Findings After a Nuclear Accident: Three Mile Island

Laura Davidson, Ph.D.
Andrew Baum, Ph.D.

*T*he potential for human-made catastrophes always exists, and it has been argued that such events are inevitable (Perrow 1984). The most serious nuclear power accident in the United States occurred in Pennsylvania at the Three Mile Island (TMI) nuclear reactor. This event provided us with the opportunity to study the psychological and physiological consequences of exposure to nuclear-related catastrophes. In this chapter we discuss the event, the circumstances surrounding the accident, and its effect on the community. We also present the results of a long-term follow-up study of residents living near the damaged reactor.

Three Mile Island

In mid-1968, a relatively unnoticed but ultimately important event occurred: Metropolitan Edison was granted the construction permit for the Three Mile Island Nuclear Power Station near Harrisburg, Pennsylvania. The plant was to consist of two reactors. The first, Unit 1, was completed and placed on-line in 1974. Over the next few years, several radioactive leaks were reported, but no major problems occurred. Unit 2 was dedicated in 1978, shortly before the new year. Like Unit 1, Unit 2 experienced problems from the time it went on-line until a major accident occurred there on March 28, 1979, just 3 months after the unit became operational (Starr and Pearman 1983).

The accident was the result of a series of mechanical and human errors. The reactor was designed to shut down automatically when a pump taking cooling water to the core of the reactor stopped working. This occurred as the accident began, and at the same time a pressure relief valve opened as it should have. However, the valve stuck and remained open. Water that was supposed to cool the reactor core flowed through the open valve, threatening the level of coolant water in the reactor. At the same time, an operator shut the auxiliary water pumps down. The gauge that would have told the operators that the pressure relief valve was stuck open was located on a control panel that was not visible to the staff.

As a result of these events, the level of water in the reactor dropped dramatically, exposing the core and generating great heat. Equipment and fuel rods melted, fused, and may have exploded. In 1985, when investigators were able to examine the extent of the damage fully, it appeared that core temperatures had reached 5,000°F and that 50% of the fuel in the core had melted. Some experts believe that the reactor was within 30 minutes from melting through the reactor vessel when cooling water was finally restored (Peterson 1989).

Although the accident occurred in the early morning hours on March 28th, the public was not notified of the accident until later that morning. Initial news releases were assurances that no radiation had been released. Throughout the day, area residents were told that little or no radiation had been released, but later in the afternoon, the governor's office announced that Metropolitan Edison had provided misleading information. Residents were then told that the accident was more serious than had been suggested and that radiation had been released.

The following day, little new information was provided, but on the 30th the situation continued to worsen. First, the governor advised residents living within 10 miles of the plant to remain inside, with doors and windows closed. Two hours later, he recommended that pregnant women and preschool children living within 5 miles of the plant evacuate the area.

The evacuation advisory remained in effect until April 9th, marking an end to the emergency period that immediately followed the accident. This established a 2-week period of threat and disruption for people living near TMI, and it appears certain that this period was stressful. At least three major aspects of the situation contributed to this stress: the potential danger, the information crisis, and the evacuation warnings (Starr and Pearman 1983).

The Community Surrounding the Reactor

The community of Middletown is a small town in south central Pennsylvania, near Harrisburg. In the mid-1960s, growth in the communities surrounding TMI was able to bolster the local economy. A new Harrisburg Airport was built, the Pennsylvania State University located its Capitol Campus in the area, and the TMI power station provided jobs for many area residents. Before the accident, the plant was viewed positively by most area residents because it replaced an outdated coal-fired power plant.

Houts et al. (1988) described the characteristics of the community within a 5-mile radius of the reactor and compared them with national norms. In July 1979, they used random-digit dialing to collect data from a total of 692 people. These data were then compared with 1980 United States census data. There were no differences in age of heads of households or family size. There were fewer blacks, area residents were slightly better educated (more had finished high school), and more area residents had incomes over $10,000 a year than the nation as a whole. These data suggest that residents living within 5 miles of the plant tended to be of slightly higher socioeconomic status than other United States residents.

Impact of the 2-Week Emergency Period

Although no studies were conducted during the first few days of the emergency period, there is evidence to suggest that the emergency period was stressful for area residents. As noted earlier, the governor recommended that pregnant women and preschool children living within 5 miles of the plant evacuate. However, the actual number of evacuees suggested more widespread concern. It was estimated that as many as 144,000 people living within a 15-mile radius of the plant evacuated (Hu and Slaysman 1984). Within a 5-mile radius of the plant, evacuation estimates ranged from 50% to almost 70% of the population (Houts et al. 1988). The mean length of time that people stayed away from the area was 4–5 days, and more than half the people who evacuated traveled more than 30 miles (Houts et al. 1988). The most common reason cited for evacuation was that the situation seemed dangerous (Flynn 1979; Flynn and Chalmers 1980). Other reasons given for leaving included the fear of an evacuation order and distress due to conflicting information (Flynn 1979). Of the people who stayed, reasons cited included faith in a deity, lack of ability to leave, inability to leave a job, fear of looters, and not viewing the situation as dangerous (Flynn 1979).

There is other evidence that stress responding increased immediately after the accident. The use of alcohol, tobacco, sleeping pills, and tranquilizers increased after the accident (Houts et al. 1980). Physicians also reported more somatic complaints and higher blood pressures after the accident (J. Leaser, unpublished observations, 1979). Nearby residents reported more upset and demoralization, they perceived the accident as threatening to their health, and they reported greater distrust of authorities (Dohrenwend et al. 1979).

Subgroups of the population did not exhibit the same degree of distress. For example, although adults typically reported more upset and demoralization, power plant workers showed little evidence of this pattern of distress (Dohrenwend et al. 1979). However, junior and senior high school students exhibited distress that mirrored adult distress. Mothers with young children were particularly sensitive to stress, and one-third of these mothers reported symptoms of anxiety and depression.

Other Sources of Stress at TMI

It is undeniable that the TMI accident and 2-week emergency period that followed it were stressful for area residents. However, disasters were nothing new to the communities surrounding TMI. In 1972, Hurricane Agnes caused flooding in a large area of Pennsylvania, including the TMI area. More than one-quarter million people were forced to evacuate their homes. The area surrounding TMI was particularly affected by this storm because it lies at the confluence of the Swatara Creek and the Susquehanna River. In 1975, another tropical storm, Hurricane Eloise, dumped heavy rain on the same area, damaging property and causing residents to flee their homes. However, the nuclear accident at TMI was different and appears to have had longer effects on area residents.

After the accident at the power plant, problems continued to plague the TMI residents. The information problems, evacuation, and other aspects of the accident and emergency period caused stress, but new problems began to appear after the emergency period and probably sustained the initial stress. For example, after the accident radioactivity periodically leaked from the damaged reactor. Excess radiation was reported in the groundwater and soil. As the cleanup of the damaged reactor continued, radioactive canisters traveled by truck in and out of the surrounding communities. This movement carried the threat of an accident that would again release radioactivity. These cleanup activities continued until late 1989, when the damaged reactor was slated to enter monitored storage.

In addition, local newspapers carried stories about an increase in infant hypothyroidism. If these reports were accurate, the disease could have been related to exposure to radioactive iodine at the time of the accident. Newspapers also reported that the infant mortality rate was higher than normal in the 6 months after the accident within a 10-mile radius of the plant. Although the validity of these two stories was subsequently denied, many residents fear that they will never know the truth because others accused that the denials were part of a cover-up (Starr and Pearman 1983).

In addition to these reports that periodically punctuated the newspapers, two major community stressors occurred after the accident. In July 1980, utility officials and officials from the Nuclear Regulatory Commission vented radioactive krypton gas, which had been trapped in the containment building since the time of the accident. This venting occurred over a 10-day period and involved direct release of radioactive gas into the environment. Also, the reopening of the undamaged reactor was hotly debated, and Unit 1 was finally put back on-line in October 1985 (General Public Utilities 1988). Adding to these problems were concerns about harm that many residents believed had already been done because radiation can cause diseases such as cancer, which may take years to become detectable. Many residents may have worried about these long-term consequences about which they could do very little.

Stress Beyond the Emergency Period

Because of the continuing cleanup, the controversy that surrounded the restart of Unit 1, and ambiguity about the possible long-term stress effects related to low-level radiation exposure, most experts agree that sources of threat remained for area residents long after the initial crisis. At least 25% of the population reported that they still felt threatened by the power plant 5 months after the accident (Flynn and Chalmers 1980). Houts et al. (1980) evaluated residents in July 1979 and again in 1980, 9 months after the accident. In telephone interviews, they continued to find evidence of elevated distress 9 months after the accident, including loss of appetite, overeating, trouble sleeping, feeling shaky, trouble thinking clearly, irritability, and anger. Bromet (1980) interviewed mothers of preschoolers after the accident and again 9 months later. Although symptom reporting decreased between her first and second interview, it was still elevated relative to control levels at both times. Dohrenwend et al. (1979) also reported long-term distrust of authorities after the accident, probably related to the poor and often contradictory information provided by responsible officials during the crisis.

Two research groups continued to study this situation beyond a year after the accident. Bromet and her research group conducted a series of studies on several different groups (e.g., Bromet and Dunn 1981; Bromet et al. 1982; Dew et al. 1987a). They studied mothers of preschool children from the time of the accident until the restart of Unit 1 in 1985. In general they reported that mothers had elevated levels of anxiety and depression in the year after the accident as well as 32 and 42 months later. They also reported that the restart of Unit 1 in 1985 was associated with more symptoms when compared with data collected between 2 and 3 years after the accident (Dew et al. 1987b). Another program of research on TMI has focused on symptoms of stress in a small sample of area residents and controls (Baum et al. 1983b; Davidson and Baum 1986; Davidson et al. 1982; Fleming et al. 1982; Schaeffer and Baum 1984). These studies began 15 months after the accident, when the Nuclear Regulatory Commission was considering plans to vent the radioactive krypton gas that had been trapped in the containment building since the accident. This began a longitudinal study assessing stress symptoms at approximately 6-month intervals for 5 years and then annually for 5 more years.

The original research design included four groups. One consisted of residents living within a 5-mile radius of TMI. The other three groups were control groups. One was made up of people living about 80 miles away from TMI and approximately 15 miles from any power plant (Frederick, Maryland). The other two groups were composed of people living within 5 miles of two power plants: one an undamaged nuclear power plant (Oyster Creek, New Jersey) and the other a traditional coal-fired power plant (Dickerson, Maryland). These groups were intended to provide information about potential stress associated with living near any power station.

Quasi-random sampling procedures were used to recruit subjects. Neighborhoods in each of these four areas were selected on the basis of demographic comparability. Streets within these communities were then randomly selected, and every third house on a street was approached. If the person answering the door was an adult, he or she was recruited as a participant in the study. Approximately 70% of the people approached agreed to participate, and there were no differences in response rate among the four groups. Informed consent was obtained, and subjects were paid for their participation.

In 1982, two of the control groups were dropped: the group living near the undamaged nuclear reactor and the group living near the coal-fired power plant. These groups did not differ from the group living in Frederick, and subject attrition made continuing to follow them impractical.

The original focus of the study was to evaluate the effect of the venting of the krypton gas that was trapped in the containment building at the time of the accident. For this reason, subjects were interviewed four times in 1980: 3–5 days before the venting of the krypton gas in July, 7 days after the venting began, 3–5 days after the venting, and, finally, 6 weeks after the venting was completed. Subjects were then assessed once or twice a year until 1989.

A multilevel research strategy was used to assess stress in these groups. This involves simultaneous assessment of psychological, behavioral, physiological, and biochemical indicators of stress. Self-reported symptoms of stress were assessed with the Symptom Checklist 90—R (Derogatis 1977). This scale can be used to provide a total symptom reporting score as well as measures of somatic distress, anxiety, depression, suspicion, fear, alienation, hostility, interpersonal difficulties, and concentration deficits. Subjects were asked how much they were bothered by 90 different symptoms over a 2-week period. Other affective measures of stress included the Beck Depression Inventory (Beck et al. 1961). Intrusive and avoidance thinking were assessed using the Horowitz Impact of Events (Horowitz et al. 1979). Mediators of stress were also evaluated, including perceived control, extent of social support, and coping strategies.

Behavioral changes that accompany stress may be assessed in several different ways. Performance measures are based on the notion that stress will affect motivation, concentration, or persistence, or other factors that might influence performance before, during, or after exposure to a stressor. Although behavior was assessed in several ways at TMI, a proofreading task derived from laboratory studies of stress (Glass and Singer 1972) proved to be the most consistent indicator of stress. Therefore, proofreading performance was assessed regularly among these subjects. The task consisted of a seven-page passage in which errors were systematically inserted. Errors included typographical errors, spelling errors, punctuation errors, and so on. Subjects were asked to read the passage and to circle each error that they found. They were given 5 minutes to complete this task.

Physiological indicators of stress included elevation of subjects' resting heart rate and systolic and diastolic blood pressure. Subjects were asked to relax for 15 minutes, and at the end of that period three measures of heart rate and blood pressure were taken and averaged. In addition, estimates of sympathetic nervous system activity were obtained by assaying subjects' urine for the hormones epinephrine and norepinephrine. These hormones vary as a function of exposure to stress (Frankenhaeuser 1975). To obtain long-term estimates of sympathetic activity, subjects were asked to provide urine over 15-hour collection periods. They were asked to void urine into a specimen container to which a noncaustic preservative was added. Urine was collected between 6 P.M. and 9 A.M. to avoid disruption of normal daily activities. A small sample was saved and frozen for later assay (Durrett and Zeigler 1980).

Persistence of Stress

The lingering effects of the TMI situation were clear during the first 5 years after the accident. Through 1984, TMI area residents as a group reported more bothersome symptoms than did subjects serving as controls. These differences were consistent for total symptom reporting as well as the individual subscales of the Symptom Checklist 90—R. TMI subjects also performed more poorly on the proofreading task, finding fewer of the inserted errors. These results suggest that TMI subjects were exhibiting stress-induced concentration or motivation deficits. Biological indicators of stress also indicated that TMI area residents were experiencing chronic stress. People living near TMI had significantly faster heart rates and higher systolic and diastolic blood pressures than control subjects. Over time, TMI subjects consistently excreted more norepinephrine in their urine than did controls. This pattern of results was similar for epinephrine; however, the differences between the groups were not always statistically significant.

The pattern of results began to change in 1985. In 1985, TMI subjects continued to report more somatic complaints, they performed more poorly on the proofreading task, and they exhibited higher blood pressure and excreted more catecholamines in their urine than control subjects. However, other self-reported symptoms of distress were no longer significantly different from those of controls. Davidson et al. (1991) proposed several reasons for the lack of symptom reporting in the presence of performance and physiological changes. Perhaps the most simple explanation was that subjects were no longer bothered by the symptoms. Like people who experience elevated levels of arousal at all times, TMI residents may be blunting affective experience (Schachter 1971). Alternatively, subjects might have adapted to their situation, causing chronic stress to diminish. In fact, many physical symptoms were no longer present; it may just take longer for biological and behavioral changes to disappear.

Follow-up data suggested that subjects had learned to cope with their stressful experiences or that the degree of threat present in the environment had decreased. Data collected in 1988 and 1989 indicated that the TMI and control groups no longer differed on any of the stress measures. With time, residents may have become more confident in their ability to prevent another accident or their ability to minimize the consequences of prior exposure. When the undamaged reactor was restarted without any problems, people may have become more confident as well. We found no evidence that the restart caused any additional stress among area residents (Davidson et al. 1991). As time passed and residents remained relatively healthy, they may have become less worried about the risks associated with possible low-dose radiation exposure. By the late 1980s, many of the earlier sources of threat were gone. Much of the radioactive contamination had been removed or otherwise disposed of, and it was estimated that the damaged reactor would be placed in monitored storage by the end of 1989.

Mediators of Stress

Although these data showed that as a whole TMI subjects exhibited more symptoms of stress compared with control subjects, not all TMI subjects exhibited these symptoms of stress. However, these differences were not based on demographic differences. One reason for the differential impact may be related to the way subjects coped with the situation. To assess coping, the Ways of Coping Inventory (Folkman and Lazarus 1980) was administered. Subjects were asked to indicate which of 68 ways of coping they used to deal with problems. The scale contained subscales that measure emotion-focusing coping and problem-focusing coping.

Data showed that for TMI residents, use of more emotion-focused coping was associated with fewer symptoms of stress than less use of this type of coping (Collins et al. 1983). On the other hand, subjects using a lot of problem-focused coping exhibited more symptoms of stress than subjects using this coping strategy less. The stress levels of control subjects did not vary as a function of either type of coping strategy (Baum et al. 1983a).

The reason that emotion-focused coping was more effective for TMI residents was probably related to features of the accident and ensuing situation. There was little that individual residents could do to avert the accident, and once the accident occurred citizen groups seemed relatively ineffective in altering policy. Although residents could do little when it came to the power plant, they could alter their emotional responses to the events. Once coping was successful, self-esteem would be enhanced, and residents would have greater perceptions of control. These feelings of control would then lessen the impact of the stress (Collins et al. 1983).

Social support may also play an important role in responding to stress. Research suggests that during stressful periods people benefit from social relationships (e.g., Cohen and McKay 1984). There are two basic theories related to the benefits of social support. The first assumes that high levels of social support are of benefit regardless of the presence of stress. Alternatively, the "stress buffering" hypothesis suggests that social support is beneficial only during periods of stress. When stress is absent, social support has no influence on background levels of stress (Cohen and McKay 1984).

A six-item social support scale was administered to examine the relationship between social support and stress responding in the TMI and control groups (Fleming et al. 1982). Overall, results suggested that having little social support was associated with more stress-related problems for the TMI group. That is, TMI subjects with the lowest social support scores reported the most overall symptoms and more alienation, depression, and anxiety. These subjects also performed the most poorly on the proofreading task. TMI subjects reporting higher levels of social support did not exhibit the same stress symptoms. The level of social support did not influence these measures for the control subjects. However, the pattern of findings for TMI area residents differed for somatic distress and catecholamine excretion. TMI subjects, regardless of the level of social support, reported more symptoms and excreted more epinephrine and norepinephrine in their urine. Also, independent of group, higher levels of social support were associated with fewer catecholamines and less somatic distress. Fleming et al. suggested that somatic distress and catecholamine excretion may reflect measures of arousal that may be less responsible to the benefits of having social support. Although social support may influence stress responding to the extent that it is less aversive (overall symptom reporting may decrease, and behavioral deficits may be less severe), it may not be sufficient to ameliorate stress responding completely.

Interventions

Although intervention strategies were not tested among residents living near TMI, these data provided us with some insight into what might be effective ways of alleviating stress. Strategies that promote "healthful" styles of coping and strategies that enhance social supports should be effective.

These data suggest that for TMI residents, emphasis on stress management and emotion-focused coping may be a good way of reducing stress. Coping strategies in general are probably most effective when they enhance perceptions of control (Baum et al. 1983a). As suggested earlier, in situations such as at TMI, where direct action was relatively ineffective, it may be most beneficial to focus on managing one's emotional response. Although concerned citizens should not be discouraged from taking action because of the potential for greater good, it may be less personally beneficial to cope with some stressors in this way. If, for example, residents discover that a nearby factory has been leaking hazardous chemicals, short of moving, they may decide on several courses of action. Some residents may fight the company. These people may eventually stop the company from releasing hazardous chemicals, but it could take years to accomplish this goal. When these residents are fighting the company, they are likely to experience more stress than uninvolved residents. As noted, data collected among TMI residents suggested that those with problem-focused coping styles exhibited more symptoms of stress. However, if this action-oriented group succeeds, their neighborhood may become a safer place to live. Other people may reappraise the situation and decide that the chemicals are really not that dangerous. Although these people will not exhibit the same distress as some of their neighbors, they are more likely to continue to live in an unsafe environment. Denial or reappraisal may work best in acute situations. As long-term problems drag on and become more difficult to ignore or reinterpret, these strategies may break down. Thus, when promoting a coping strategy, it is important to take into account the particular situation, how effective the coping strategy will be, and long-term goals.

Also from our TMI data it is clear that social support may be a powerful mediator of stress. Solomon (1985) described ways in which mental health workers may enhance social support in disaster victims, suggesting that social support networks should be both strengthened and built. The most effective policy would use professionals, para-professionals, and family members to create or enhance such networks. On an organizational level, available resources should be assessed. The media could be used to promote the use of resources. Community members could be trained to detect problems and make referrals. Finally, promoting activities with preexisting neighbors and friends would be important. In addition, new support groups could be formed.

Conclusions

With the abundance of technology in our world today, it is important that mental health professionals are aware of the types of events that are likely to lead to long-term stress responding. Situations that involve exposure to chronic environmental hazards may be particularly detrimental. These situations pose long-term threats, influence perceptions of control, and create uncertainty and unpredictability.

The accident at TMI provided us with a unique opportunity to study long-term responding to a technological disaster. From this work, it is clear that technological disasters may be associated with chronic stress in some people. However, not everyone will be affected by the situation in the same ways. Furthermore, there are some mediators of the stress that may be enhanced by psychological interventions. As a caveat to this, however, Fleming and Baum (1985) suggested that it may not be in victims' best interest to eliminate stress responses completely. In some instances, stress responses may be viewed as vital to self-preservation since they prepare an organism to deal with adversity and motivate it to prevent further occurrences that may involve threat.

References

Baum A, Fleming R, Singer JE: Coping with victimization by technological disaster. Journal of Social Issues 39:117–138, 1983a

Baum A, Gatchel RJ, Schaeffer MA: Emotional, behavioral and physiological effects of chronic stress at Three Mile Island. J Consult Clin Psychol 51:565–572, 1983b

Beck A, Ward C, Mendelson M, et al: An inventory for measuring depression. Arch Gen Psychiatry 42:667–675, 1961

Bromet E: Preliminary Report on the Mental Health of Three Mile Island Residents. Pittsburgh, PA, Western Psychiatric Institute, University of Pittsburgh, 1980

Bromet EJ, Dunn L: Mental health of mothers nine months after the Three Mile Island accident. Urban and Social Change Review 14:12–15, 1981

Bromet E, Schulberg HC, Dunn L: Reactions of psychiatric patients to the Three Mile Island nuclear accident. Arch Gen Psychiatry 39:725–730, 1982

Cohen S, McKay G: Social support, stress and the buffering hypothesis: a theoretical analysis, in Handbook of Psychology and Health, Vol 4. Edited by Baum A, Singer JE, Taylor SE. Hillsdale, NJ, Lawrence Erlbaum, 1984, pp 253–267

Collins DL, Baum A, Singer JE: Coping with chronic stress at Three Mile Island: psychological and biochemical evidence. Health Psychol 2:149–166, 1983

Davidson LM, Baum A: Chronic stress and post-traumatic stress disorders. J Consult Clin Psychol 54:303–308, 1986

Davidson LM, Baum A, Collins D: Stress and control-related problems at Three Mile Island. Journal of Applied Social Psychology 12:349–359, 1982

Davidson LM, Weiss L, Baum A: Acute stressors and chronic stress at Three Mile Island. Journal of Traumatic Stress 4:481–494, 1991

Derogatis LR: The SCL-90 Manual I: Scoring, Administration, and Procedures for the SCL-90. Baltimore, MD, Clinical Psychometrics Unit, Johns Hopkins University School of Medicine, 1977

Dew MA, Bromet EJ, Schulberg HC: A comparative analysis of two community stressors' long-term mental health effects. Am J Community Psychol 15:167–184, 1987a

Dew MA, Bromet EJ, Schulberg JC, et al: Mental health effects of the Three Mile Island nuclear reactor restart. Am J Psychiatry 144:1074–1077, 1987b

Dohrenwend BP, Dohrenwend BS, Kasl SV, et al: Report of the Task Group on Behavioral Effects to the President's Commission on the Accident at Three Mile Island. Washington, DC, U.S. Government Printing Office, 1979

Durrett LR, Zeigler MG: A sensitive radioenzymatic assay for catechol drugs. J Neurosci Res 1980, pp 587–598

Fleming R, Baum A: The role of prevention in technological catastrophe. Prevention in Human Services 4:139–151, 1985

Fleming R, Baum A, Gisriel MM, et al: Mediation of stress at Three Mile Island by social support. Journal of Human Stress 8:14–22, 1982

Flynn C: Three Mile Island Telephone Survey: Preliminary Report on Procedures and Findings. Seattle, WA, Social Impact Research, Inc., 1979

Flynn C, Chalmers J: The social and economic effects of the accident at Three Mile Island (NUREG/CR-1215). Washington, DC, U.S. Nuclear Regulatory Commission, 1980

Folkman S, Lazarus RS: An analysis of coping in a middle-aged community sample. J Health Soc Behav 21:219–239, 1980

Frankenhaeuser M: Experimental approaches to the study of catecholamines and emotion, in Emotions: Their Parameters and Measurements. Edited by Levi L. New York, Raven, 1975, pp 202–234

General Public Utilities: Chronology of Significant Events. New Jersey, Communications Department, General Public Utilities, 1983

Glass DC, Singer JE: Urban Stress: Experiments on Noise and Social Stressors. New York, Academic Press, 1972

Horowitz M, Wilner N, Alvarez W: Impact of Events Scale: a measure of subjective stress. Psychosom Med 41:209–218, 1979

Houts PS, Miller RW, Tokuhata GK, et al: Health-related behavioral impact of the Three Mile Island nuclear incident. Report submitted to the Three Mile Island Advisory Panel on Health Research Studies of the Pennsylvania Department of Health, Part I, April 8, 1980

Houts PF, Cleary PD, Hu TW: The Three Mile Island crisis: psychological, social and economic impacts on the surrounding population. University Park, PA, The Pennsylvania State University Press, 1988

Hu TW, Slaysman KS: Health-related economic costs of the Three Mile Island accident. Socioeconomic Planning and Science, 1984, pp 183–193

Perrow C: Normal Accidents: Living With High Risk Technologies. New York, Basic Books, 1984

Peterson C: The continuing clean-up: 1 billion and counting. The Washington Post, March 28, 1989, pp A1, A8

Schachter S: Emotion, Obesity and Crime. New York, Academic Press, 1971

Schaeffer MA, Baum A: Adrenal cortical response to stress at Three Mile Island. Psychosom Med 46:227–237, 1984

Solomon SD: Enhancing social support for disaster victims, in Disasters and Mental Health: Selected Contemporary Perspectives (DHHS Publ No ADM 85-1421). Rockville, MD, U.S. Department of Health and Human Services, 1985, pp 107–121

Starr P, Pearman W: Three Mile Island Sourcebook, Annotations of a Disaster. New York, Garland, 1983

Index

SETON HALL UNIVERSITY
McLAUGHLIN LIBRARY
SO. ORANGE. N. J.